The Nightingale
Model of
Nursing

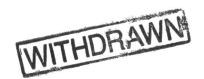

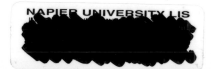

The Nightingale
Model
of Nursing

Rob van der Peet

Ph.D., M.Phil., B.D., S.R.N., R.N.T.

Campion Press, Edinburgh

1995

British Library Cataloguing in Publication Data:

Peet, Rob van der
Nightingale Model of Nursing
I. Title
610.7301

ISBN 1 873732 11 2

Published by Campion Press
384 Lanark Road, Edinburgh EH13 0LX

Designed and typeset in 10/12pt Palatino by Artisan Graphics, Edinburgh

Printed and bound by Bell & Bain, Glasgow

Contents

Contents

Introduction

By common consent the publication of *Notes on nursing* (Nightingale, 1859b)[1] and the founding of the Nightingale training school for nurses in 1861, heralded the beginning of modern nursing. However, these historical events reveal little or nothing about the Nightingale model of nursing: the model which is said to have marked 'the beginning of the development of theoretical models of nursing' (Riehl & Roy, 1974, p. 16). To grasp the meaning of this model (encompassing Nightingale's concepts of nursing, nursing education and professional nursing) requires an analysis of the model's

- presuppositions (a remarkable mixture of statistical inquiry, religious speculation and zeal for social reform); and,
- implications (a sanitary approach to nursing).

These presuppositions and implications have been at the source of the historical events which made up her life. Given these presuppositions and implications, questions arise as to whether the Nightingale model of nursing justifies Nightingale being regarded as the founder of modern nursing and to what extent this model has influenced the conceptual development of nursing. The answers to these questions emerge from the detailed analysis of Nightingale's concepts of:

- nursing;
- nursing education;
- professional nursing; and,
- the practical application of her concept of nursing.

The analysis put forward here breaks new ground insofar as it is aimed at clarifying Nightingale's impact on later models of nursing, particularly

---

1 The text referred to here is reproduced as an appendix.

in the United States, by means of a conceptual interpretation rather than by a reconstruction of the chronology of the historical events which made up her life. It will therefore focus primarily on Nightingale's views as they have been handed down in her writings, viz.:

- *Notes on nursing* (1859b),
- *Nurses, training of* (1882a) and *Nursing the sick* (1882b),
- *Sick nursing and health nursing* (1893).

As far as the conceptualisation of nursing is concerned it will become clear that, because of the religious presuppositions and the sanitary implications of the Nightingale model of nursing, Nightingale should not be regarded as the founder of modern nursing. Moreover, between them, these presuppositions and implications have given the Nightingale model of nursing a flavour so idiosyncratic as to be prohibitive of exercising any influence at all. This is not to say that Nightingale should not be awarded the title of 'founder of modern nursing', only that it should be attributed to her for reasons other than the model of nursing which bears her name.

I: *Florence Nightingale: the person and her work*

The person

Florence Nightingale (1821–910) was born in Italy on 12th May, 1820, while her parents were visiting the city of Florence. Her parents named her after the place of her birth. As a well-educated and sophisticated young woman, she was immersed in the social circles of upper middle class Victorian England. However, claiming to have had a calling from God, she turned her mind to more serious concerns. In 1851 she went to Kaiserswerth in Germany where, as an alternative to the Catholic nursing orders, the Lutherans had established an order of Deaconesses who were trained to nurse and provide welfare support for the sick and needy. Following this early initiation into nursing, she returned to London and eventually became superintendent of the Institute for the care of Sick Gentlewomen in Distressed Circumstances.

In 1854 Nightingale led a party of nurses to Scutari to care for the sick and wounded in the Crimean War. The dreadful sanitary conditions and what she perceived as their direct influences on health had a powerful impact on Nightingale; she herself contracted 'Crimean fever' (probably typhoid fever). On her eventual return to England she continued her commitment to nursing and combined this with an intensive campaign for sanitary reform. These were to be the main concerns of the remainder of her life.

Despite constant ill-health and exhaustion, she continued to write prolifically on nursing and sanitation throughout the 1850s. The years 1859–1861 were particularly significant, as it was in this period that she founded the Nightingale School of Nursing at St Thomas's Hospital in London. Here she introduced what is commonly recognised as the first secular training for nurses.

Throughout her life, Nightingale remained a single woman, apparently given at various times to excesses of mood and severity, and seldom in perfect good health herself. She was an intense and driven person by nature and devoted herself to her various causes with tenacity and stubbornness. Apart from a close relationship with Richard Monckton Milnes, later Lord Houghton, while in her late teens and early twenties, Nightingale had no close emotional ties outside her family and few close acquaintances. She died in London on 13th August, 1910.

It is generally claimed that Nightingale is the founder of modern nursing. However, to assess more precisely the influence she has exerted on the conceptual development of nursing is difficult, mainly because of the way nursing historians have presented both her life and her writings on nursing. As to the Nightingale model of nursing, it should be added that nursing historians are evidently inclined to consider it (if they consider it at all) in isolation from Nightingale's endeavours in other areas, notably religion and statistics. This approach may result in a more or less comprehensive chronology of historical events but it is not conducive to a good understanding of the Nightingale model of nursing, let alone an accurate appraisal of its significance for the conceptual development of nursing.

The biographies

Florence Nightingale's life has given rise to virtually as many different interpretations as the number of her biographers. The first biography of lasting importance was 'The life of Florence Nightingale' by Cook (1913a and 1913b). It is no secret that Cook had to work within the constraints imposed upon him by the relatives of Nightingale who had commissioned this biography and wanted to see certain events, for example her love affair with Richard Monckton Milnes, kept out of the book. On the other hand, Cook must have had access to almost all of the sources available at the time because his study is still second to none as far as the documentation is concerned.

Whereas Cook, in contrast with the sentimentalised image of the lady with the lamp still dominant at his time, painted a more or less detached picture of Nightingale, Strachey, in his book 'Eminent Victorians', reached quite a different verdict (Strachey, 1918, p. 115):

> *Everyone knows the popular conception of Florence Nightingale. The saintly, self-sacrificing woman, the delicate maiden of high degree who threw aside the pleasures of a life of ease to succour the afflicted, the Lady with the Lamp, gliding through the horrors of the hospital at Scutari, and*

consecrating with the radiance of her goodness the dying soldier's couch
— the vision is familiar to all. But the truth was different. The Miss
Nightingale of fact was not as facile fancy painted her. She worked in
another fashion, and towards another end; she moved under the stress of
an impetus which finds no place in the popular imagination. A Demon
possessed her. Now demons, whatever else they may be, are full of interest.
And so it happens that in the real Miss Nightingale there was more that
was interesting than in the legendary one; there was also less that was
agreeable.

Apparently, it was Strachey's iconoclastic interpretation that has given a
new lease of life to the traditional semi-mythical image which antedated
Cook's biography, resulting in a new wave of biographies in which
Nightingale was depicted alternatively as, for example, the lost com-
mander, the soldiers' heroine, the fiery angel, the angel of the Crimea or
the lady with the lamp (Hebert, 1981). The third most influential biography has been written by Woodham-Smith (1951) who followed Cook's
chronology of events as well as Strachey's interpretation of Nightingale's
personality.

More recently published studies on Nightingale's life, on the other hand,
tend to be less comprehensive than these biographies. In turn, they
provide a greater in-depth view of particular aspects of her life like her
ailments since the return from the Crimea (Pickering, 1974), her use of her
reputation and power (Smith, 1982), or her influence on nursing and
nursing education (Prince, 1982; Baly, 1984). Whereas the comprehensive
biographies were based upon the groundwork done by Cook and portrayed Nightingale as the intelligent, masterful, soft-spoken lady with the
lamp, these studies are based upon original research of the historical
sources and tend to present a far less idealised image of Nightingale.

Finally, special mention should be made of the study by Kalisch and
Kalisch (1983a and 1983b) concerning the sentimentalised images of
Nightingale presented by popular biographies, stage productions, film,
radio and television dramatisations. To sum up, it appears that more than
half a century after Nightingale's death, nursing historians have finally
reached the stage at which it is possible to publish well documented and
relatively unbiased studies of certain aspects of her life.

The original works
As far as Nightingale's original works are concerned, the situation shows
some striking similarities. Except for Cook's study, which deals with her
writings in more detail than any other biography, the interest shown by

most nursing historians has been limited to 'Notes on nursing' (Nightingale, 1859b), her first book on nursing which has always been readily available. A notable exception is Newton's dissertation 'Florence Nightingale's philosophy of life and education' (1949) but, regrettably, this study is buried in the library of Stanford University and has never been published. Fortunately, the content has been reported extensively by Barritt (1973).

Newton's study reflected the growing interest in Nightingale's writings at the time. In 1949, the National League of Nursing Education thought it fit to publish 'Nursing of the sick', the report of the International Congress of Charities, Correction and Philanthropy which met in Chicago during the World's Fair in 1893. This report included Nightingale's 'Sick nursing and health nursing' (Nightingale, 1893), which was her last comprehensive and authoritative statement on the nature of nursing.

In 1954, Seymer's 'Selected writings of Florence Nightingale' was published. This compilation contained, amongst others, 'Nurses, training of' (Nightingale, 1882a) and 'Nursing the sick' (Nightingale, 1882b), two articles which Nightingale later contributed to Quain's 'A dictionary of medicine', (Quain, 1895).

Consequently, Nightingale's most important writings on nursing have become more accessible. The same cannot be said about her other writings, or as Bishop reportedly put it (Bishop & Goldie, 1962, p. 5):

> *The popular legend of Florence Nightingale is being perpetuated, while her own writings are neglected, and her most important achievements forgotten. There is little understanding of her real message for today. ... It was her friend Benjamin Jowett who wrote of Miss Nightingale that she had become a legend in her own lifetime. She remains a "legend" - but for all the wrong reasons.*

This situation, however, was about to change as a result of a research project which started in 1955 and was initiated and sponsored by the International Council of Nurses (ICN) and the Florence Nightingale International Foundation (FNIF). This project has resulted in 'A biobibliography of Florence Nightingale', (Bishop & Goldie, 1962), and 'A calendar of the letters of Florence Nightingale' (Goldie, 1980). As a result of Bishop's and Goldie's efforts, Nightingale's original works have become more readily available (Goldie, 1987; Poovey, 1991; Vicinus & Nergaard, 1989; Skretkowicz, 1992 and 1993).

Towards a reappraisal of Florence Nightingale

Focus

The foregoing review goes a long way to show that, whereas, at present, nursing historians have at their disposal the historical sources needed to study Florence Nightingale's life and writings, the sheer volume of these sources — amounting to some 200 books, pamphlets and articles, and more than 15,000 letters — has made it virtually impossible to cover them all. It seems likely, therefore, that nursing historians will refrain from writing comprehensive biographies and confine themselves to the study of particular aspects of her life and works.

So far, however, this change of emphasis has contributed hardly anything to resolve the controversy perpetuated by the semi-mythical and the iconoclastic images of Nightingale. On the contrary, it seems rather to have prompted a debate more intense than ever before. Whereas, for example, Cook is accused of playing down the frictions between Nightingale and her mother and sister, Woodham-Smith is said to magnify them (Kalisch & Kalisch, 1983a).

Other issues are whether Nightingale happened to be a lesbian (Gordon, 1978) or not (Palmer, 1983a), if she suffered from physical and mental disease (Palmer, 1983a) and if she used her illness to her own advantage (Pickering, 1974).

Apart from these more or less anecdotal issues, the controversy is concerned with issues relevant to the present time, like the acclaimed independence of the Nightingale training school for nurses. This controversy, incidentally, also exposes a line of division between researchers of American and English origin.

American researchers (e.g. Stewart, 1944; Newton, 1949) tend to portray the Nightingale school's educational independence as the hallmark of professional education. After the introduction of the so-called Nightingale system of nursing education in the United States its independence, so the interpretation goes, was lost because, at an early stage, hospitals and doctors gained control over the training of nurses, resulting in an apprenticeship type of training.

On the other hand, Prince (1982) and Baly (1984), both English researchers, have convincingly demonstrated that the original Nightingale school never achieved any educational independence whatsoever. Their research shows that, in fact, it was only a matter of years after the school's foundation in 1860 before the hospital governors and the medical profession were effectively in control of the training of the Nightingale nurses. Whereas these researchers blame Nightingale for this failure, the American researcher Palmer (1983b), although acknowledging Nightingale's failure, attempts to explain it away by pointing to a whole range of mitigating circumstances.

The Nightingale school's educational independence therefore appears to be based upon myth rather than reality. But, whereas the English researchers, because of the present problems in nursing education which can be traced back to the failure of the Nightingale system, would prefer to tackle these problems by facing the reality of Nightingale's failure rather than upholding the myth of her educational reform, American researchers make no secret of the nursing profession's 'vested interest in preserving Florence Nightingale's reputation and in promoting the positive association evoked by her name. ... Her value and fame ought to be used for the advancement of the profession and not shelved as out-of-date' (Kalisch & Kalisch, 1983b, p. 278).

As for Nightingale's original works, American researchers have demonstrated a similar attitude by taking her writings at face value and using them as it suited their own purposes (e.g. Roberts, 1937; Stewart, 1931; Thompson, 1980). By publishing 'Nursing of the sick' in 1949, for example, American nursing leaders deliberately used Nightingale's contribution politically to support their struggle for the professional education of nurses.

One promising approach would be to investigate the Nightingale model of nursing in relation to two other subjects in which Nightingale showed so much interest, viz. religion and statistics. Cook (1913a, p. 428) has characterised her as a 'passionate statistician', and there is hardly a better way of putting her interest in religion and statistics into perspective. From these interests, in combination with her activities in the field of nursing, an essentially different Nightingale emerges — the religiously inspired woman, advocating the need of statistical inquiry which was to result in practical applications such as sanitary nursing. This characterisation, if considered further, indicates the need for a new interpretation of the Nightingale model as well as a reappraisal of its significance for the conceptual development of nursing.

Religion
Nightingale's passion for statistics might be attributed to her religious beliefs as she has expressed them in 'Suggestions for thought' (Nightingale, 1860a, 1860b, and 1860c). She had started writing on religion as early

as 1852 but did not finish the three volumes until 1860. Who can better sum up the content of the 800+ octavo pages of this work than Nightingale herself, in a letter to her father (in: Cook, 1913a, p. 482):

> I think the subject is this: Granted that we see signs of 'universal law' all over this world, i.e. law or plan or constant sequences in the moral and intellectual as well as physical phenomena of the world – granted this, we must, in this universal law, find the traces of a Being who made it, and what is more of the character of the Being who made it. If we stop at the superficial signs, the Being is something so bad as no human character can be found to equal in badness, and certainly all the beings He has made are better than Himself. But go deeper and see wider, and it appears as if this plan of universal law were the only one by which a good Being could teach His creatures to teach themselves and one another what the road is to universal perfection. And this we shall acknowledge is the only way for any educator, whether human or divine, to act – viz. to teach men to teach themselves and each other. If we could not depend upon God, i.e. if this sequence were not always to be calculated upon in moral as well as in physical things — if He were to have caprices (by some called grace, by others answers to prayers, etc.) there would be no order in creation to depend upon. There would be chaos. And the only way by which man can have Free Will, i.e. can learn to govern his own will, to have what will he thinks right (which is having his will free), is to have universal Order or Law (by some miscalled Necessity). I put this thus brusquely because philosophers have generally said that Necessity and Free Will are incompatible. It seems to have appeared to God that Law is the only way, on the contrary, to give man his free will. And this I have attempted to prove. And further that this is the only plan a perfectly good omnipotent Being could pursue.

In Nightingale's writings, there are few words which figure so prominently as the word 'law', or for that matter, 'universal law', and understandably so, for it was the most basic assumption of her whole argument, that (Nightingale, 1860a, p. 3):

> observation and experience afford evidence that law is manifested in the beginning, the constitution, the history, and the tendency of all modes of being that have a beginning.

By the manifestations of law, Nightingale meant specific 'uniformities in nature', so-called 'laws' of nature', which expressed 'uniform relations of simultaneity and succession, in which one mode of being is observed to exist to another' (Nightingale, 1860a, p. 10). As for every mode of being which had a beginning, so she reasoned, it was possible to pinpoint its constituent elements (Nightingale, 1860a, pp. 10–14):

- its *beginning,* which 'is uniformly preceded by and simultaneous with certain conditions, without which it is true to say of each existing mode of being which has had a beginning that it would not have begun; while, if ever or whenever these conditions recur, the same mode of being will again begin to be.'

- its *constitution* or *nature,* '...something in which indiviuals uniformly resemble each other, so as to admit of being classed together; or ... definite states uniformly simultaneous with or successive to definite antecedent or co-existing circumstances in beings of the same class or in an individual.'

- its *history,* which 'is in accordance with law –*i.e.*– from that time present in which a mode of being begins to be, in each successive time present some change takes place; all such change being relative to a definite nature or constitution in the being in which it takes place, as well as to its circumstances of simultaneity and succession to other modes of being.'

- its *tendency* or *future,* meaning that all modes of being which have a beginning 'are throughout existence tending to some definite state or mode of being – *i.e.* the present is a definite preparation for a definite future.'

What all these uniform relations add up to is that, given a mode of being which, for example, is called 'being ill', and assuming that no treatment is given, it is possible to pinpoint the environmental circumstances which have caused the illness, its symptoms, its progress as well as its result. If, on the other hand, treatment is started by manipulating the environmental circumstances affecting this mode of being, it should likewise be possible to point out the resulting mode of being's constituent elements. These elements, therefore, indicated the existence of a universal law which not only presupposed a law-giver, i.e. God, but implied a deterministic view of man too. An important corollary of this conclusion is that the way Nightingale described the constituent elements of these modes of being made them susceptible to statistical inquiry (Cook, 1913a, p. 480):

The laws of God were, she held, discoverable by experience, research, and analysis; or, as she sometimes put it, the character of God was ascertainable, though his essence might remain a mystery. The laws of God were the laws of life, and these were ascertainable by careful, and especially by statistical, inquiry.

This was also the point where the free will of man, to be analysed shortly, entered into the discussion.

Statistics

Whereas remarkably little is written about Nightingale's religious views, except for Cook (1913a and 1913b), Tarrant (1914) and Mantrip (1932), her endeavours in the field of statistics have generated a wider interest (Kopf, 1916; Nutting, 1929; Agnew, 1958; Grier & Grier, 1978; Diamond & Stone, 1981). It is beyond doubt that Florence Nightingale has contributed as much to statistics as to nursing, if not more so, also taking into account that she was elected to fellowship in the Royal Statistical Society in 1858 and made an honorary member of the American Statistical Society in 1874. The major part of her statistical research was concerned with sanitation (e.g. Nightingale, 1859a).

As to the origin of Nightingale's interest in statistics there are two conflicting explanations. According to Cook (1913a) and Kopf (1916) her interest was inspired by the book 'Sur l'homme et le développement de ses facultés, ou essay de physique sociale', published in 1835 and written by Adolphe Quetelet, the Belgian statistician whom she once described as the 'founder of the most important science in the whole world' (Agnew, 1958, p. 665). The other explanation, put forward by Diamond and Stone (1981), holds that it was her association with Dr. Farr and other leading statisticians in England which was at the source of her interest in statistics. Moreover, she knew only the second edition of Quetelet's book, entitled 'Physique sociale' which he had given to her in 1869. Otherwise, Diamond and Stone (1981, p. 71) argue, she would not have requested him in 1872 to publish a second edition on the grounds that the first edition was unobtainable in England.

Notwithstanding this controversy, it is beyond doubt that Quetelet's work influenced Nightingale deeply. One of the things that must have appealed to her in Quetelet's work was his belief that the causal explanation of human behaviour, for example criminal behaviour, had to be looked for in the antecedent and coexistent conditions of behaviour observed and that, insofar as statistics could be used to display the regularities of this behaviour, such a social phenomenon became material for scientific inquiry (Grier & Grier, 1978, p. 104). In these so-called 'moral statistics' Nightingale must have seen the confirmation of:

> her deep conviction, variously expressed in her several papers, that the social and moral sciences are in method and substance statistical sciences. ... Statistics, she mused, discovered and codified law in the social sphere

and thereby revealed certain aspects of the 'character of God'. (Kopf, 1916, p. 98)

In other words, by means of statistics Nightingale could deal not only with physical but moral modes of being too, thereby adding a new dimension to her statistical research, viz. the laws of moral behaviour manifesting God's law which, as she wrote to her father, was 'the only way — to give man his free-will' The germ from which Nightingale's religious philosophy is said to have been developed was, as she herself once put it (Cook, 1913a, p. 479):

God's scheme for us was not that He should give us what we ask for, but that mankind should obtain it for mankind.

In her opinion, the laws of nature reflected God's (Nightingale, 1860a, pp. 5–6):

will, that a definite mode of being should invariably be simultaneous with certain definite (and invariably the same) circumstances.

More importantly, it was also God's will that (Nightingale, 1860a, pp. 7, 8):

.. man is capable of finding out what state and what circumstances will be SIMULTANEOUS. And thus, within certain limits, he may determine his state.

Between them, these statements on God's dealings with man were tantamount to the antithetic relationship between necessity manifested in God's law, on the one hand, and man's free will exemplified by his reason, feeling, conscience, and all his other faculties, on the other.

The synthesis Nightingale attempted to arrive at was that 'human will accords with law' which was her somewhat idiosyncratic interpretation of the atonement or, as she used to spell it, the 'at-one-ment' (Nightingale, 1860a, p. 40), resulting in the 'union of God and man in one common thought, feeling, purpose' (Nightingale, 1860a, p. 9).

Because man was part of nature, Nightingale considered him to be subject to God's laws or the 'laws of nature'. Given a certain constitution affected by certain environmental circumstances, man therefore always acted according to God's 'laws of nature', in that:

His moral and His physical law stand on exactly the same basis: neither is ever broken: bodies do not fall upwards; and His moral law which says 'if you kill, certain consequences will follow, and if certain circumstances take place, you will kill,"'is always kept. (Nightingale, 1860b, pp. 303–304)

To discover the character of God, man had to 'study the nature of God in other natures, in which He has manifested and revealed His own' (Nightingale, 1860b, p. 271), stressing that 'not phenomena, but laws, are the only evidence of character. We cannot estimate a man's character from any action which he performs, but only from the principles which govern his whole conduct. So with God' (Nightingale, 1860b, p. 79). On the other hand, Nightingale was painfully aware that, in order to find out God's law, 'People do not ... investigate physiological laws, consult statistics, or make out what they can from the experiences of those who have experience' (Nightingale, 1860b, p. 217). This was one of the greatest frustrations she experienced during her campaigns for sanitary reforms.

The study of physical and moral phenomena, advocated by Nightingale, was based upon the assumption that 'The whole of the laws of God is such that they are self-rectifying, with regard to their effect upon man's well-being' (Nightingale, 1860a, p. 6). If, for example, a person became ill, it was not God who was to blame for inflicting disease upon him, but the person's ignorance or indifference with regard to His laws. Given that God's law was always being kept and man was afforded both the inducement (being ill) and the means (sanitary science) to discover the uniform relations manifesting His law, God had enabled him to 'advance in [the] knowledge, will, [and] power' (Nightingale, 1860a, p. 17) needed to improve his health. These human capabilities were to return in Henderson's definition of nursing (Henderson, 1966). The study of uniform relations in the state of the body to decide whether man's mode of being was healthy or unhealthy was more or less subordinated to the study of similar relations in the state of the mind determining whether man was morally right or morally wrong (Nightingale, 1860b, p.44):

> We cannot be good in all circumstances. God does not intend it; and this, instead of making us do nothing, is the greatest spur we can have to exertion. If God does not intend us to be right under such and such circumstances, we must alter them.

It is from remarks like these that the deeper significance of Nightingale's writings can be inferred. Although she admittedly emphasised the need for scientific inquiry into the laws of nature to justify sanitary reform, such reform also required a moral decision for or against such reform.

Given, however, that she held man's moral mode of being to be subject to the laws of nature which determined the uniform relations between his moral condition and the environmental circumstances affecting it, he could not possibly be free to decide one way or another. Her position therefore appeared to be based upon a circular reasoning. In order to break the resulting deadlock, she would emphasise that (Nightingale, 1860c, pp. 78–79):

Mankind has to learn by experience, 1st, what are his capabilities? 2nd, what are all the various laws of God concerning them? 3rd, that it is desirable to cultivate these capabilities aright; 4th, which of these laws enable him to do so? 5th, how to keep them? 6th, how to incline himself to keep them? All this man has to learn and to practice before he can be one with God.

Finally, sanitation was just one of the many areas in which this process of learning by experience had to take place (Nightingale, 1860a, p. 50):

Sanitary science is showing how we may affect the constitution of the living and of future lives. In one direction, sanitary science is understood to apply to the physical nature; but each part of man's nature affects every other. Moreover, there is a sanitary science essential to each of man's faculties and functions. For each there is an appropriate state and operation – in other words, a healthy state; and there is a science discoverable as to how, by what means to bring about that appropriate state.

It was thus by virtue of God's laws always being kept, that man was afforded his free will (albeit a freedom of choice rather than absolute free will) to choose for or against approximating his union with God's thought, feeling, and purpose. The major lesson to be learnt from this was that man, instead of being at the mercy of circumstances, was 'in the hands of God' (Nightingale, 1860b, p. 46). For all the necessity manifested in God's laws, man's free will enabled him to approximate the union with God, if only he was willing to use the inducement and the means afforded to him, and this in itself amounted to a moral decision in favour of social reform (Nightingale, 1860b, p. 267):

A true understanding of the nature of God and man, of our relations to God and to our fellow-creatures, depends upon, requires the right exercise of, the whole nature of all mankind. We can only have such right exercise by a right organization of society, by mankind arranging circumstances so that they will have employment, work, suited to their natures, suited to call forth their natures into right exercise.

In summary, just like the laws of God revealed His government of the world, mankind had to learn how to govern its own behaviour according to these laws in order to become one with God. This process of learning involved:

- observation by means of statistics,
- reflection as to the lesson to be learnt from it, and
- social reform.

The relatively new science of statistics therefore provided Nightingale with the scientific vindication of her religious beliefs (Nightingale, 1860b, p. 346):

> *Our religious creed consists in this — belief in an omnipotent eternal spirit of love, wisdom, righteousness, manifesting itself by calling into existence, by definite laws, beings capable of the happiness of love, wisdom, and righteousness, — capable of advancing themselves and each other in divine nature – living in an universe in which, by definite law, the means and inducement are afforded which insure their advance through their own activity to humanity's blessedness. Observation, reflection, experience are that which furnishes the evidence.*

Towards a positive theology

Nightingale's interest in religion and statistics influenced each other to the degree that, between them, they enabled her (Nightingale, 1873a) to defend her concept of God as a God of law, whose character may be learnt from social and moral science (Cook, 1913b, p. 218):

> *against some current ideas of Christian churches on the one side, and against the too cold and impersonal creed, as she thought, of Positivism on the other.*

The article in Fraser's Magazine, cited here by Cook, was a condensed version of the far more extensive inquiry of these issues in 'Suggestions for thought' which prompted Nightingale to develop a new 'positive theology' (Nightingale, 1860c, pp. 178–202), already foreshadowed by her remarks earlier in that year (Nightingale, 1860a, p. 35):

> *Wiser than former generations in abstaining from futile speculation, some powerful minds show a determination to seek no truth except what is supposed to admit of proof. We conceive that the limit to our inquiry should be those subjects on which we can hope progressively to receive evidence.*

Nightingale's positive theology was based upon 'the revelation of moral evidence' (Nightingale, 1860a, p. 115) rather than the revelation through the Bible, or through the church, or through both of them: 'Now we say that there is a revelation to every one, through the exercise of his own nature – that God is always revealing Himself' (Nightingale, 1860b, p. 95). In her view, this openness to empirical reality signalled a new phase in theology which was antedated by the miraculous theology and the supernatural theology in which God was associated with miracles and special providences respectively. According to Nightingale's 'positive' theology, however '... we see Him in law. But law is still a theology, and the finest' (Nightingale, 1860b, pp. 155–156).

Nightingale's positive theology was also directed against 'the conscientious unbelievers' of her day, especially the positivist philosopher Comte, who said that 'when all is said and done, and the whole of the faculties exercised, &c., all that we can discern with these faculties is the law of nature', an attitude which elicited the following rhetorical questions 'Is there not an absurdity in saying that all we can discern is whatever is, is according to law? For is it not our experience of law that it always springs from a will, from a purpose?' (Nightingale, 1860c, p. 26).

Thirteen years later, she attacked Huxley for having said that 'Objects of sense are more worthy of your attention than your inferences and imaginations' by emphasising that 'the finest powers man is gifted with are those which enable him to infer from what he sees what he can't see. They lift him into truth of far higher import than that which he learns from the senses alone' (Nightingale, 1873a, p. 568).

Most importantly though, Nightingale's positive theology provided her with the foundation of a moral science which she described as '... the science of the social and political improvement of man, the science of educating and administering the world by discovering the laws which govern man's motives, his moral nature', or the study of the character of God, 'because the laws of the moral world are the expressions and solely the expressions of the character of God' (Nightingale, 1873a, p. 577).

Whereas Bacon and Newton had laid the foundation for physical science by discovering the method by which all enquiry into physical science had to be conducted to be successful, she believed she had found an equally successful method for moral science, viz. careful observation by means of statistics. Between them, these sciences were inevitably to lead to social reform (Nightingale, 1873a, p. 575):

> In the very measure of the progress we make in finding out the real facts of moral science, e.g. educational science, or the real facts of physical science, e.g. sanitary science, in that very measure those facts show the perfect God leading man on to perfection. ... Exactly as we find out the real facts, we find that every one of those facts has attached to it just the lesson which will lead us on to social improvement.

This parallelism between physical and moral science was a recurring theme in Nightingale's writings, exemplified, amongst others, by her admiration for social improvements as a result of advances in physical science which she sought to copy in the field of morality (Nightingale, 1860b, p. 39):

> *Suppose that we had done with steam as we have done with morals, that is, asserted that "everything has been discovered, nothing more is to be done, you have only to believe;" should we have had any railroads, any steamboats, any manufactures? yet within the last thirty years how astounding has been the advance?*

Another example is provided by her repeated comparisons between the 'uniform' differences in the state of the body (healthy versus unhealthy), on the one hand, and those of the mind (morally right versus morally wrong) on the other. These comparisons, however, did not stop her from using the word 'healthy' also to identify 'the healthy state of mind', or 'moral feeling', i.e. 'the consciousness, existing with a feeling of satisfaction in the right, of dissatisfaction in the wrong' (Nightingale, 1860a, p. 14).

In both cases, however, the 'uniform' differences to be discovered manifested law for they existed relatively to the 'uniform' conditions of man's bodily and mental state. As for the former, these differences existed 'relatively to physical organization and to circumstances which affect it', while as for the latter, they existed 'relatively to physical organization and to circumstances which otherwise definitely and uniformly affect the state of mind' (Nightingale, 1860a, pp. 12–13). The wording used by Nightingale herself reflected her own assessment of the state of the art at the time of both physical and moral science.

It is worth noting that Nightingale's positive theology, most poignantly advocated in her first article in Fraser's Magazine (Nightingale, 1873a), amounts to the position that both religion and science are meaningful to the degree that they result in social reform. In this sense, she can be seen as a 'pragmatist avant la lettre', a fact first perceived by Cook (1913a, p. 488):

> *Miss Nightingale was broad-minded in her attitude towards creeds and churches. For her own part she believed that religious truth was positive, and could be discovered; but in her outlook upon the beliefs of others, she judged them by their fruits. ... There is a school of philosophy, much current in our day, which carries this point of view further. The meaning of a conception, it tells us, expresses itself in practical consequences, if the*

conception be true; religious truth is relative to the individual; the way to test a religion is to live it.

It is this religious pragmatism which calls for a renewed interpretation of the Nightingale concept of nursing as well as a reappraisal of its historical significance for the conceptual development of nursing.

Florence Nightingale: founder of modern nursing?

Given Nightingale's religious pragmatism, it remains to be seen to what extent it has influenced her concepts of nursing, nursing education and professional nursing (Nightingale, 1859b, 1882a and 1882b, 1893). Her religious pragmatism does not immediately become apparent when reading her original writings on nursing. The first impression gained from these writings is that they demonstrate a good deal of common sense, soundly based upon her detailed observation and her rich experience, and, even when turning a blind eye to the many references to God, Nature and the laws of nature, her line of reasoning does make sense. If these references are taken into account, however, a rather different image of Nightingale emerges from her texts, namely that of the religious pragmatist who attempts to become one with God by discovering His laws and adapting her own will, and that of others as well, to His will.

On reading Nightingale's main works on religion (Nightingale, 1860a, 1860b, 1860c, 1873a, and 1873b) it became apparent that her religious beliefs played a most important role in her writings on nursing to the effect that, without the former, the latter would not have been written in the first place. For reasons explained earlier, and because only 150 copies of 'Suggestions for thought' (Nightingale, 1860 a, b and c) have been printed, these original works on religion have become far less widely known than her writings on nursing. Apart from that, these writings make difficult reading as Nightingale omitted to edit 'Suggestions for thought' as carefully as her writings on nursing, with the effect that she repeated herself time and again. Moreover, in discussing her personal beliefs, she compared them with those of others who may have been well known in her day but are not any more.

All this goes a long way to explain why few biographers have attempted an interpretation of her writings on nursing in the light of her original works on religion such as will be undertaken here. Clarifying the interrelationships between Nightingale's views on religion and nursing is necessary in order to assess her real influence on the conceptual development of nursing. As a result, it will become clear why Nightingale should not be regarded as the founder of modern nursing.

II: Nightingale's concept of nursing

Nursing and nature

'Notes on nursing' (Nightingale 1859b) is said to contain Nightingale's principles or philosophy of nursing (Seymer, 1954) and rightly so, because it deals primarily with sanitary nursing, the concept of nursing which she never abandoned. The edition referred to throughout this book is the more widely available original 1859 edition of 'Notes on nursing'. There were at least three versions of the book produced between 1859 and the mid-1870's and not all of these got into print or were widely available. The most definitive version was that known as the second version published in 1860 (see Skretkowicz, 1992). This was in fact an enlarged version produced particularly for those serious readers who would require a definitive reference work on nursing. However, this second version was not in fact widely available until a definitive edition based on it, revised and with additions, was produced by Skretkowicz (1992) in the work referred to above. Skretkowicz's admirable edition is perhaps the most authoritative extant source of 'Notes on nursing' and the interested reader is referred to this text. However, given the still more readily available original 1859 version, references to and quotations from 'Notes on nursing' in this book refer specifically to that edition, and it is reproduced here as an appendix.

At the time of writing 'Notes on nursing' Nightingale was highly optimistic about the growing importance of sanitary science (Nightingale, 1859b, p. 3):

> *Every day sanitary knowledge, or the knowledge of nursing, or in other words, of how to put the constitution in such a state as that it will have no disease, or that it can recover from disease, takes a higher place. It is recognized as the knowledge which every one ought to have — distinct*

from medical knowledge, which only a profession can have.

By distinguishing two different kinds of knowledge to combat disease, she also suggested two different notions of disease, in the medical and in the sanitary meaning of the word, and it was the latter rather than the former which she considered relevant for nursing. A book such as 'Notes on nursing', she believed, was needed because she thought it was extraordinary that (Nightingale, 1859b, p. 7, see also 1893, pp. 29–30):

whereas what we might call the coxcombries of education — e.g. the elements of astronomy — are now taught to every school-girl, neither mothers of families of any class, nor school-mistresses of any class, nor nurses of children, nor nurses of hospitals, are taught anything about those laws which God has assigned to the relations of our bodies with the world in which He has put them. In other words, the laws which make these bodies, into which He has put our minds, healthy or unhealthy organs of those minds, are all but unlearnt. Not but that these laws – the laws of life – are in a certain measure understood, but not even mothers think it worth their while to study them — to study how to give their children healthy existences. They call it medical or physiological knowledge, fit only for doctors.

By comparing the laws of astronomy and the laws of life she added a moral dimension to her concept of nursing. This interpretation is vindicated by her use of the example of astronomy in 'Suggestions for thought' too (Nightingale, 1860b, p. 202):

In astronomy, Copernicus, Galileo, Kepler, Newton, Laplace, Herschel, and a long line of saviours, we may call them, if we will – discoverers they are more generally called, – have saved the race from intellectual error, by finding out several of the laws of God. ... In the same way, there may be, there must be saviours from social, from moral error.

It is this comparison between the physical and moral dimension of man's existence, reflected in the manifold comparisons between medicine and nursing, which casts a new light on Nightingale's view of the nature of nursing. This interpretation is further vindicated by her definition of nursing (Nightingale, 1859b, p. 75):

And what nursing has to do ... is to put the patient in the best condition for nature to act upon him.

This definition which links nursing with nature, and thereby with the laws of nature and consequently with God's will, rather than with medicine, she never abandoned (e.g. Nightingale, 1893, p. 26). Underlying her concept of nursing was her view of man's relationship to God being mediated by his experience and observation of natural phenomena manifesting God's universal law, the foundation of her religious pragmatism. This assumption which was at the source of so many of her endeavours can be illustrated by her explanation as to the cause and the nature of disease.

Miasmatism versus contagionism

One of the major issues in health care during the last century was the scientific explanation of epidemic diseases. According to the contagionist theory, diseases originated from infectious matter which was transmitted from one person to another. This causal explanation of disease was based upon the so-called germ theory which emerged during the 1860s. For reasons explained below, Nightingale never accepted this theory.

On the other hand, according to the miasmatic theory, diseases were the result of harmful influences in the environment which were called miasmas or miasmatas, although it proved to be rather difficult to pinpoint the 'mechanics of the miasmatic theory, whether the inhalation of putrescent substances oxidised and corrupted the bloodstream, or whether the exhalations of such substances or affected persons introduced poisons into neighbouring bodies' (Smith, 1982, p. 98).

Notwithstanding its lack of explanatory power, the theory of miasmatism gained much support during the first half of the nineteenth century. Nightingale is said to have held this belief since at least her Harley Street days (early 1850s), when she had probably acquired it from Chadwick and other sanitarians' writings in the 1840s (Smith, 1982, p. 98), while in 'Notes on hospitals' she pointed to medical evidence in a translation of Paulus Aegineta corroborating her sanitary observation and experience (Nightingale, 1859a, p. 6, footnote).

Contrary to what Smith (1982, p. 98) and Strachey (1918, pp. 168–169) would lead us to believe, speculations about the mechanics of the miasmatic theory were not completely foreign to Nightingale's nature (Nightingale, 1858, pp. 128–133):

> It is a vulgar error to suppose that epidemics are occasioned by the spread of disease, from person to person, by infection or contagion; for it is an ascertained fact that, before any people is attacked epidemically, the disease attacks individuals in a milder form, one at the time, at distant intervals, for weeks or months before the epidemic appears. Before an epidemic of cholera, these cases consist generally of diarrhoea of more or less intensity, followed by a rapidly fatal case or two, very much resembling cholera. ...

Experience appears to show that without this antecedent preparatory stage, affecting more or less the entire population of a town or district, the occurrence of an epidemic is impossible – the epidemic being, in fact the last or, so to speak, the retributive stage of a succession of antecedent phenomena extending over months or years, and all traceable to the culpable neglect of natural laws. It is simply worse than folly, after the penalty has been incurred, to cry out "contagion," and call for the establishment of sanitary cordons and quarantine, instead of relying on measures of hygiene. Epidemics are lessons to be profited by: they teach, not that "current contagions" are "inevitable" but that, unless nature's laws be studied and obeyed, she will infallibly step in and vindicate them, sooner or later.

In sharp contrast with other sanitarians, however, Nightingale based her speculations not only upon observation and experience but upon her religious beliefs too, for when it came to the reason for holding these views, she asked herself what lesson either contagion or infection contained as to the image of God (Nightingale, 1873a, pp. 575–576):

- *contagion* 'Were "contagion" a fact, what would be its lesson? To isolate and to fly from the fever and cholera patient, and leave him to die; to kill the cattle; instead of improving the conditions of either. This is the strictly logical "lesson" of "contagion." If it is not strictly followed, it is only because men are so much better than their God. If "contagion" were a fact – this being the lesson which it teaches – can we escape the conclusion that God is a Spirit of Evil, and not of Love?'

- *infection* 'Now take the real facts of "infection." What is their lesson? Exactly the lesson we should teach, if we wanted to stir man up to social improvement. The lesson of "infection" is, to remove the conditions of dirt, of over-crowding, of foulness of every kind under which men live. And even were not socalled "infectious" disease attached to these conditions by the unchanging will of God, it would still be inseparable from social improvement that these conditions should be removed. Disease is Elijah's earthquake, which forces us to attend, to listen to the "still small voice." May we not therefore say that "infection" (facts and doctrine) shows God to be a God of love? And this is but one instance.'

These speculations, based upon observation and experience, were typical of Nightingale's religious pragmatism to the effect that, whereas miasmatism entailed practical lessons as to which circumstances God wanted man to change, contagionism did not.

Apart from that, contagionism presupposed for every infectious disease a first case, directly infected by God. Given her belief in God's wisdom and benevolence, she therefore could not but accept the miasmatic explanation of disease. Not surprisingly, Strachey (1918, p. 167) has therefore characterised Nightingale's image of God as being that of a 'glorified sanitary engineer' in which it is hard to distinguish between 'the Deity and the Drains.'

Nightingale's speculations on the causal explanation of disease adds a moral or religious significance to some of her seemingly purely scientific statements on nursing like 'That there is no such thing as "inevitable" infection, is the first axiom of nursing' (Nightingale, 1882b, p. 337), or 'The fear of dirt is the beginning of good nursing' (Nightingale, 1882b, p. 344). She was convinced that her sanitary approach, if taken to its logical conclusion, would result in a situation in which 'Scarlet fever and measles would be no more ascribed to "current contagion," or to "something being much about this year," but to its right cause; nor would "plague and pestilence" be said to be "in God's hands," when, so far as we know, He has put them into our own' (Nightingale, 1893, p. 30).

On the other hand, she was well aware of the growing body of opinion, also based on observational evidence, which supported the contagionist view, but, even if confronted with empirical data contradicting her miasmatic point of view, Nightingale could not bring herself to change her mind. This shows that her religious belief, more than anything else, was the yardstick by which she evaluated the results of observation and experience, thereby raising the level of the discussion from a physical to a moral level, and this, as has been shown earlier, was the core of her religious pragmatism. Similar observations can be made when it comes to her views on the nature of health and disease.

Health and disease

Nature
'Notes on nursing' starts with some very significant assumptions as to the nature of disease which not only reflect Nightingale's religious pragmatism but are essential to grasp the meaning of her concept of nursing too (Nightingale, 1859b, p. 5):

> *Shall we begin by taking it as a general principle – that all disease, at some period or other of its course, is more or less a reparative process, not necessarily accompanied with suffering: an effort of nature to remedy a process of poisoning or of decay, which has taken place weeks, months,*

sometimes years beforehand, unnoticed, the termination of the disease being then, while the antecedent process was going on, determined?

This notion of disease was clearly inspired by Nightingale's stance on the controversy between miasmatism and contagionism, affected as it was by her religious pragmatism. To prove her point, as might be expected from her, she first appealed to observation (Nightingale, 1859b, p. 5):

In watching disease, ... the thing which strikes the experienced observer most forcibly is this, that the symptoms or the sufferings generally considered to be inevitable and incident to the disease are very often not symptoms of the disease at all, but of something quite different – of the want of fresh air, or of light, or of warmth, or of quiet, or of cleanliness, or of punctuality and care in the administration of diet, of each or of all of these.

In 'Notes on hospitals' she put it even more poignantly when she related that, on the basis of her observation of hospital wards, it was impossible for her 'to resist the conviction that the sick are suffering from something quite other than the disease inscribed on their bedticket' (Nightingale, 1859a, p. 3). In Nightingale's opinion, suffering as a result of disease had thus to be distinguished from suffering due to the lack of the right circumstances affecting man's healthy mode of being. However, if asked 'Is such or such a disease a reparative process? Can such an illness be unaccompanied with suffering? Will any care prevent such a patient from suffering this or that?' she humbly answered 'I do not know' (Nightingale, 1859b, p. 6). But what she did know was what kind of practical action was needed to answer these questions decisively (Nightingale, 1859b, p. 6):

... when you have done away with all that pain and suffering, which in patients are the symptoms not of their disease, but of the absence of one or all of the above-mentioned essentials to the success of Nature's reparative process, we shall then know what are the symptoms of and the sufferings inseparable from the disease.

From these remarks it can be inferred that, in Nightingale's opinion, the suffering accompanying disease was a moral or religious rather than a sanitary issue, for it is worth noting here that Nightingale wrote 'Nature' and not 'nature.' This was the way she used to refer to 'the Absolute and Perfect Moral Nature, from whom, through the law which reveals His existence and all that we can comprehend of His nature, we may attain enlightenment possible to us concerning the right' (Nightingale, 1860a, p. 31). She therefore appears to have favoured a theological rather than a medical notion of health and disease. Moreover, her opinion as to how to deal with the suffering of the sick also exposes another characteristic of her religious thinking – her optimism, based upon God's plans for man, that, ultimately, at one time or another in the future, the battle against disease could be won, for (Nightingale, 1892, p. 33):

> ... after all it is health and not sickness that is our natural state – the state that God intends for us. There are more people to pick us up when we fall than to enable us to stand upon our feet. God did not intend all mothers to be accompanied by doctors, but He meant all children to be cared for by mothers.

It was this line of reasoning which also came to the fore in her writings on nursing analysed here (Nightingale, 1859b, pp. 6–7; 1893, p. 24). Granted this theological interpretation of Nightingale's notions of health and disease, it goes without saying that the analysis has to start with her notion of disease.

Disease

To return to the suffering accompanying disease, in 'Suggestions for thought' this phenomenon did not seem to pose a problem to Nightingale at all. On the contrary, she seemed even to welcome it (Nightingale, 1860b, p. 237):

> In certain diseases there is no remedy known for acute and constant suffering, and it is right that it should be so, in order to bring about circumstances in which the causes of such suffering shall be removed, in which man shall attain a right physical state.

The practical implications of the suffering of the sick, indicated here, were matched by those of disease (Nightingale, 1882b, pp. 334–335):

> Sickness or disease is Nature's way of getting rid of the effects of conditions which have interfered with health. It is Nature's attempt to cure – we have to help her.

In 'Sick nursing and health nursing' Nightingale repeated this definition of disease, only adding that 'Diseases are, practically speaking, adjectives, not noun substantives' (Nightingale, 1893, p. 26). The meaning of this somewhat cryptic statement had been explained by her as early as 1859 (Nightingale, 1859b, p. 19, footnote):

> Is it not living in a continual mistake to look upon diseases, as we do now, as separate entities, which _must_ exist, like cats and dogs? instead of looking upon them as conditions, like a dirty and a clean condition, and just as much under our own control; or rather as the reactions of kindly nature, against the conditions in which we have placed ourselves.

This explanation of the nature of disease suggests that Nightingale considered the mode of being which was called 'disease' to be subject to the laws of God which 'visit us with consequences till we do something. We may try the experiment; we may sit still if we like; but, while we do so, God's laws will never cease molesting us. His laws have provided that it shall be impossible to us – that our nature is such, our desires, energies, inclinations such, that we can't do nothing' (Nightingale, 1860b, p. 168).

In other words, disease and the suffering accompanying it, however physically real to the person concerned, were the phenomena from which he was to discern the laws of God so that he could let his will accord with God's law. These phenomena therefore pointed to some moral or religious reality behind or underlying the reality observed and experienced by the sick – the will or the character of God. As for the practical lessons to be learnt from disease, Nightingale was very adamant (Nightingale, 1859b, pp. 17–18):

> And now, you think these things [pure air, pure water, efficient drainage, cleanliness, and light] trifles, or at least exaggerated. But what you 'think' or what I 'think' matters little. Let us see what God thinks of them. God always justifies His ways. While we are thinking, He has been teaching. I have known cases of hospital pyaemia quite as severe in handsome private houses as in any of the worst hospitals, and from the same cause, viz., foul air. Yet nobody learnt the lesson. Nobody learnt _anything_ at all from it. They went on _thinking_ – thinking that the sufferer had scratched his thumb, or that it was singular that 'all the servants' had 'whitlows,' or that something was 'much about this year; there is always sickness in our house.' This is a favourite mode of thought – leading not to inquire what is the uniform cause of these general 'whitlows,' but to stifle all inquiry. In what sense is 'sickness' being 'always there,' a justification of its being 'there' at all? ... Yet nobody learns the lesson. Yes, God always justifies His ways. He is teaching while you are not learning. This poor body loses his finger, that one loses his life. And all from the most easily preventible causes.

This text illustrates Nightingale's writings on nursing to be susceptible to two different interpretations. Taken at face value it seems to stress the need for sanitary reform, but it also suggests a more important lesson to be learnt – the character of God and His way of dealing with man. This theological interpretation of Nightingale's writings on nursing is vindicated by her religious works. In 'Suggestions for thought', for example, she contrasted the physical and moral laws of God to the effect that people do not mind being saved by the former, while, as to the latter, 'Most people have not learnt any lesson from life at all – suffer as they may, they learn nothing, they would alter nothing – if they began life over again they would live exactly the same life as before' (Nightingale, 1860b, pp. 202–203).

Health

The theological interpretation of Nightingale's definition of disease is further vindicated by her definition of health (Nightingale, 1882b, pp. 334–335; see also 1893, p. 26):

Health is not only to be well, but to be able to use well every power we have to use.

This definition should be taken to mean that being healthy was not limited to the absence of disease in the medical meaning of the word but also assumed man's 'capability to find out how to bring about right physical being – right circumstances in which to live' (Nightingale, 1860c, p. 55). From the way Nightingale has defined the word 'power' in 'Suggestions for thought' it can be inferred that her definition of health indeed had a theological meaning for her (Nightingale, 1860b, pp. 53–54):

Man has capability to learn how circumstances regulate and modify human nature, to learn what circumstances develop and exercise human nature aright. By the united efforts of mankind, in accordance with God's ever-present, ever-efficient law, to bring about such circumstances is man's work. The capability for this is man's power.

The implications for nursing

Nightingale's view of the nature of health and disease adds a moral or religious dimension to some of her statements on nursing; for example, 'The art of nursing, as now practised, seems to be expressly constituted to unmake what God had made disease to be, viz. a reparative process' (Nightingale, 1859b, p. 6), or 'To get rid of the conditions which have interfered with health is of course the first nursing step in helping Nature to get rid of the effects of those conditions' (Nightingale, 1882b, p. 337), or, 'Everything has come before health. We are not to look after health, but after sickness. Well, we are to be convinced of error before we are convinced of right; the discovery of sin comes before the discovery of righteousness, we are told on the highest authority' (Nightingale, 1893, p. 25). Nursing, as Nightingale viewed it, amounted thus to the gradual discovery and application of God's laws upon which depended whether man's mode of being was to be healthy or not, even though, at least in 1859, she was well aware of the fact that (Nightingale, 1859b, p. 6):

The very elements of what constitutes good nursing are as little under-stood for the well as for the sick. The same laws of health or of nursing, for they are in reality the same, obtain among the well as among the sick. The breaking of them produces only a less violent consequence among the former than among the latter, – and this sometimes, not always.

Nightingale used the word 'elements' here not inadvertently as she probably referred to Dalton's discovery of the system of chemical elements which she very much admired because it demonstrated the wisdom of God so well (Nightingale, 1860b, pp. 50–51). In the same way, she envisaged the discovery of the elements of man's health or of nursing, or as she is said to have put it once, 'I look forward to the day when there will be no nurses of the sick, only nurses to the well' (in: Baly, 1969, p. 2) which is consistent with her religiously inspired optimism: 'People think that the world is in the mud, and that it must stay there. We think it is in the mud too, but we are sure it is not to remain there' (Nightingale, 1860b, p. 203).

In most of her discussions on the nature of nursing, it was this religiously inspired optimism which set the tone of the argument that man, using his intelligence to discover God's laws and his free will to adopt God's will as manifested by His laws, could work out his own health by putting an end to all conditions and circumstances giving rise to disease.

Nursing: What it is, and what it is not

Sanitary nursing

Over the years, Nightingale's concept of nursing remained remarkably consistent. This is not to say that her three main publications on nursing are so identical that they are completely interchangeable. On the contrary, each one of them is directed at different readers and deals with different aspects of her concept of nursing.'Notes on nursing' (Nightingale, 1859b), for example, was 'meant simply to give hints for thought to women who have personal charge of the health of others' (p. 3), and dealt with 'sanitary nursing' as opposed to the 'handicraft of nursing' or 'surgical nursing' or 'practical manual nursing' as it was practised at the time (p. 71). In this book, Nightingale used the word 'nurse' indiscriminately for both 'amateur and professional nurses', and, whereas the latter referred to nurses of the sick and nurses of children, the former were to include friends, relations and mothers of families 'who take temporary charge of a sick person' (p. 79).

'Nurses, training of' (Nightingale, 1882a) and 'Nursing the sick' (Nightingale, 1882b), on the other hand, have been written for the probably well-educated readers of Quain's medical dictionary. Both articles were concerned with the subject of nursing in the sense of an 'art, requiring an organised practical and scientific training' (Nightingale, 1882b, p. 335) as it had been provided by the Nightingale training schools for nurses since 1861.

Finally, 'Sick nursing and health nursing' (Nightingale, 1893) stands out somewhat from the other publications on nursing as it was intended to be read by an audience of mostly professional nurses. Whereas the articles for Quain's medical dictionary had dealt with 'nursing proper, that is, nursing the sick and injured' as opposed to 'Preventive or Sanitary Nursing' and 'nursing healthy children', this publication signalled the extension of Nightingale's concept of nursing with 'health nursing' or 'general nursing' as opposed to 'nursing the sick' or 'nursing proper' and pleaded for the attention of the public to be directed to the need for the training of health-missioners as already had been done with regard to the training of sick nurses.

However, in the final analysis and despite the differences noted above, all Nightingale's writings on nursing were based on one single concept of nursing – sanitary nursing. Underlying this concept, as will emerge from the analysis of her various definitions of nursing, was her ever-present religious pragmatism rather than the opposition between medicine and nursing. Admittedly, Nightingale's works on nursing can be interpreted as an attempt to identify the differences between medicine and nursing, but her religious beliefs call for a different interpretation. For within the context of her religious pragmatism Nightingale considered medicine to be less relevant than sanitary nursing as the latter taught man about the character of God and the former did not.

'Notes on nursing'

Nightingale's sanitary approach as opposed to the medical approach, apparently already dominant at the time, comes to the fore in her first definition of nursing (Nightingale, 1859b, p. 75):

> ... *what nursing has to do ... is to put the patient in the best condition for nature to act upon him. Generally, just the contrary is done. You think fresh air, and quiet and cleanliness extravagant, perhaps dangerous,* · *luxuries, which should be given to the patient only when quite convenient, and medicine the* <u>sine qua non</u>, *the panacea. If I have succeeded in any measure in dispelling this illusion, and in showing what true nursing is, and what it is not, my object will have been answered.*

Nightingale thought these differences between nursing and medicine were so fundamental that she even considered giving her sanitary approach a new name. But, as she herself noted, she used 'the word nursing for want of a better. It has been limited to signify little more than the administration of medicines and the application of poultices. It ought to signify the proper use of fresh air, light, warmth, cleanliness, quiet, and the proper selection and administration of diet – all at the least expense of vital power to the patient' (Nightingale, 1859b, p. 6).

Table 1 Sanitary nursing and nursing proper (Nightingale, 1859b and 1882b)

Notes on nursing (Sanitary nursing)	Nursing the sick (Nursing proper)
What nursing has to do, is to put the patient in the best condition for nature to act upon him	Nursing proper means besides giving the medicines and stimulants prescribed, or applying the surgical dressings and other remedies ordered:
Ventilation and warming	The providing, and the proper use of, fresh air, especially at night - that is, ventilation, and of warmth or coolness
Light Cleanliness of rooms and walls Bed and bedding	The securing the health of the sick-room or ward, which includes light, cleanliness of floors and walls, of bed, bedding, and utensils
Petty management	
Taking food What food?	The administering and sometimes preparation of diet (food and drink)
Personal cleanliness Noise Variety Chattering hopes and advices	Personal cleanliness of patient and of nurse, quiet, variety, sympathy, and cheerfulness
Observation of the sick	Observation of the patient
Health of houses: pure air, pure water, efficient drainage, cleanliness, light	The application of remedies. In other words, all that is wanted to enable Nature to set up her restorative processes, to expel the intruder disturbing her rules of health and life. For it is Nature that cures: not the physician or nurse.

For the sake of the comparison, the sequence of the table of contents of 'Notes on nursing' has been adapted to the sequence of nursing actions in 'Nursing the sick'.

By explaining her concept of nursing and the nursing actions involved (see Table 1), Nightingale once again pointed to the difference between nursing as a derivative of medicine, on the one hand, and sanitary nursing, on the other. This raises the question of how she was to adapt her concept of nursing once the Nightingale nurses had moved into the hospital, which leads us to the definition of nursing in 'Nursing the sick' (Nightingale, 1882b).

'Nursing the sick'

In this article Nightingale understandably qualified her definition of nursing to accommodate the notion of nursing proper which included hospital nursing, private nursing, district nursing and midwifery (Nightingale, 1882b, p. 334):

> *Nursing is putting us in the best possible conditions for Nature to restore or to preserve health – to prevent or to cure disease or injury. The physician or surgeon prescribes these conditions – the nurse carries them out.*

This definition of nursing suggests a change of heart on the part of Nightingale which is not, however, borne out by the general outline of the article. On the one hand, she was admittedly very careful in awarding the physician the position he probably occupied anyway, for example, by conceding that nursing was 'the skilled servant of medicine, surgery, and hygiene' (Nightingale, 1882b, p. 335). On the other hand, she qualified this statement by emphasising that 'real nursing' existed 'in obeying the physician's and surgeon's orders intelligently and perfectly' (Nightingale, 1882a, p. 326), that is, in the nurse relying also on her own observation, reflection and training (Nightingale, 1882a, p. 323).

This diplomatic approach was probably indicated by the fact that she wrote the article for a medical dictionary and is further exemplified by her outline of the nursing actions involved. Apart from two references to the role of medicine, this outline was basically the same as the one she had given in 'Notes on nursing' (see Table 1). Moreover, in the text of the article itself it was only at the end that the relationship between medicine and nursing was mentioned. Nightingale did this by using a standard phrase to the effect that the physician, the surgeon or the medical attendant 'requires the nurse to ...', followed by those nursing actions which were the prerogative of the physician to prescribe.

Finally, she also mentioned the 'management of convalescents – a whole department of nursing in itself', and 'housekeeping' as other duties of the nurse (Nightingale, 1882b, p. 349).

'Sick nursing and health nursing'

This article is best known for the introduction of the concept of health nursing or general nursing which, while innovative in that it adopted a health promotion and home nursing perspective, covered virtually the same principles of sanitary nursing as 'Notes on nursing' (Nightingale, 1893, p. 31):

> *The work we are speaking of has nothing to do with nursing disease, but with maintaining health by removing the things which disturb it, which have been summed up in the population in general as "dirt, drink, diet, damp, draughts, drains".*

This was Florence Nightingale, the sanitary reformer, as we have come to know her from 'Notes on nursing'. Not surprisingly, she therefore saw no need to change her definition of nursing (p. 26):

> *Both kinds of nursing are to put us in the best possible conditions for nature to restore or to preserve health – to prevent or to cure disease or injury.*

Her sanitary approach to nursing also came to the fore in the nursing actions involved in both types of nursing (p. 29):

> *Nursing proper means, besides giving the medicines and stimulants prescribed, or the surgical appliances, the proper use of fresh air (ventilation), light, warmth, cleanliness, quiet, and the proper choosing and giving of diet, all at the least expense of vital power to the sick. And so, health-at-home nursing [another name used for health nursing] means exactly the same proper use of the same natural elements, with as much life-giving power as possible to the healthy.*

Even the persons practising both types of nursing remained the same. Whereas in nursing proper, it was the professional nurse who had to apply the principles of sanitation, in health nursing it was the mother of the family (p. 37). The only real innovation put forward in this paper was the introduction of a professional or trained nurse, the so-called health-missioner, who was expected to teach and instruct the mother of the family how to practise the principles of sanitation (p. 31; see also Nightingale, 1892). This conclusion is further vindicated by her comparison between sick nursing and health nursing (see Table 2).

In summing up, whereas the idea of the professional nurse in the role of the health-missioner was new, the concept of health nursing in itself amounted to nothing other than a repetition of the principles of sanitary nursing. Even Nightingale's complaints about the lack of public confidence in sanitation were repeated (p. 31):

But, in fact, the people do not believe in sanitation as affecting health, as preventing disease. They think it is a "fad" of the doctors and rich people. They believe in catching cold and in infection, catching complaints from each other, but not from foul earth, bad air, or impure water.

The same goes for the reason why she advocated this concept of nursing which, incidentally, also illustrates her persistent religious pragmatism (pp. 29–30):

The laws of God – the laws of life – are always conditional, always inexorable. But neither mothers, nor school-mistresses, nor nurses of children are practically taught how to work within these laws, which God has assigned to the relations of our bodies with the world in which He has put them. In other words, we do not study, we do not practise the laws which make these bodies, into which He has put our minds, healthy or unhealthy organs of those minds; we do not practise how to give our children healthy existences.

Conclusion

The first conclusion to be drawn is that, over the years, Nightingale's concept of nursing did indeed remain essentially the same. Her concept of sanitary nursing exemplified her optimism as to man's ability to extinguish disease and to attain a permanent state of health. Therefore, this concept (and the nursing actions involved) was more closely related to what we, at present, would call a health science rather than medical science.

More importantly, this concept of nursing was firmly based upon her religious outlook on life which gave it its typical Nightingale flavour of a morally-inspired zeal for sanitary and social reform.

This conclusion is clearly at variance with Seymer's observation that (1954, p. xi):

By 1893, a change seems to have come over Florence Nightingale's spirit. Unlike many other older women, whose ideas are incapable of expansion in later life, she saw clearly the paramount value of what one might call "preventive nursing" ... and outlines the basic principles of much that would now be classed under "public health." It was a great achievement for a woman of seventy-three, who had been out of active nursing for so many years, to have the foresight to rate prevention higher than cure.

Table 2 Sick nursing and health nursing (Nightingale, 1893).

Nursing proper (Sick nursing)	Health nursing (Health-at-home nursing)
This type of nursing was based upon a want 'nearly as old as the world, nearly as large as the world, as pressing as life or death... that of sickness.	This type of nursing was based upon the assumption that 'God did not mean mothers to be always accompanied by doctors.' Therefore there must be 'a want older still and larger still', and this was the want of being healthy (although Nightingale omitted to name it as such).
The new art created for this want was 'that of *nursing the sick*. Please mark – nursing the *sick*; and *not* nursing sickness.' This, as Nightingale pointed out, was 'one of the distinctions between nursing and medicine.' In addition, she wrote: 'We will call the art nursing proper. This is generally practised by women under scientific heads – physicians and surgeons.'	At the time, the art, as far as households, families, schools were concerned, had not yet been created, though it was an art which concerned 'every family in the world.' The art Nightingale was hinting at was 'the art of health, which every mother, girl, mistress, teacher, child's nurse, every woman ought practically to learn. But she is supposed to know it all by instinct, like a bird. Call it *health nursing* or *general nursing* – what you please. ... It is the want of the art of health, then, of the cultivation of health, which has only lately been discovered; and great organizations have been made to meet it, and a whole literature created. We have medical officers of health; immense sanitary works. We have not "missioners" of health-at-home.'
'Nursing proper means, besides giving the medicines and stimulants prescribed, or the surgical appliances, the proper use of fresh air (ventilation), light, warmth, cleanliness, quiet, and the proper choosing and giving of diet, all at the least expense of vital power to the sick.'	'And so, health-at-home nursing means exactly the same proper use of the same natural elements, with as much life-giving power as possible to the healthy.'

Table 2 *(continued)*

Nursing proper (Sick nursing)	Health nursing (Health-at-home nursing)
Nightingale omitted to mention any new science by name but, on the basis of her division between nursing proper and medicine, it can be inferred that it was certainly not medical science – it included medicine, surgery and sanitary science.	In contrast to the art, the science to meet the want of being healthy had been created but once again Nightingale did not mention it by name. However, circumstantial evidence indicates that she meant sanitary science.
The nurse proper had to be able to 'recognize the laws of sickness, the causes of sickness, the symptoms of disease, or the symptoms, it may be, not of the disease, but of the nursing, bad or good.'	Furthermore, it was upon womankind and not the nurse that the national health, as far as the household was concerned, depended. Therefore it was she, and not the nurse, who 'must recognize the laws of life, the laws of health.'
Since nursing proper was the art of nursing the sick, it could 'only be properly taught and properly learnt in the sick-room and by the patient's side.'	Sanitation could 'only be properly taught and properly learned in the home and the house.'
Nursing proper was 'to help the patient suffering from disease to live.'	Health nursing was 'to keep or put the constitution of the healthy child or human being in such a state as to have no disease.'

As a matter of fact, there was no change of heart at all as the concept of health nursing exemplified the same sanitary approach as `Notes on nursing' which had been written some 34 years earlier, except for the introduction of the professional or trained nurse as a health-missioner.

A more plausible interpretation of the course of events may be something like this. Nightingale's initial optimism as to the importance of sanitary science for the well-being of mankind had prompted her to write on the principles of sanitation and to create the Nightingale training school for nurses in order to bring about sanitary reform. During the 1860s and thereafter, however, the contagionist point of view gained more and more support, helped by the discoveries of Pasteur and many others, confirming the truth of the germ theory. During that period Nightingale's activity in the field of sanitation decreased significantly, according to

Pickering (1974) as a result of her bad health. However, in the light of her position on the controversy between miasmatism and contagionism there may well have been a second reason concerning the decreasing support for sanitary reform. After that, during the 1880s, the practice of nursing became increasingly influenced by the advances in medicine, most notably in surgery. However, at that time, too, the value of district nursing for the prevention of disease was realised, and this prompted Nightingale to seize the opportunity to reinforce her sanitary approach to nursing by introducing the concept of health nursing and the accessory health-missioner.

The second conclusion to be drawn is that Nightingale was not so much interested in the practice of nursing as in the moral lessons to be learnt from it. Her writings on nursing, it is true, contain many anecdotes and examples of the practice of nursing, both in the hospital and in the home, but she never bothered to write a comprehensive textbook of nursing. Instead, she emphasised the principles of sanitation, which she considered to be one of the major instruments by which to teach mankind about the character of God. Nursing, as she viewed it, was therefore of less importance than man's union with God. In the final analysis, using the lessons taught by sanitary observation and experience, her endeavours in the area of nursing were therefore directed at the moral improvement of mankind.

The third and perhaps most important conclusion is that the above analysis has shown Nightingale's concept of nursing to be based upon her miasmatic views as to the cause and the nature of disease. Starting with the observation of epidemic diseases, and assuming that God whom she held to be wise and benevolent could not possibly be the cause of such diseases, she arrived at the conclusion that the miasmatic explanation was the right one. As to the diseases themselves, she started with the assumption that disease was a reparative process or an effort of nature to remedy the process of poisoning or of decay, an assumption for which she found proof, time and again, in the observation of disease. Both these elements of statistical observation and religious reflection were to reappear in her concept of sanitary nursing, thereby showing that her religious pragmatism was at the source of her concept of nursing. Nightingale has not only been lauded as the founder of modern nursing but also as the founder of nurse education. This begs a question as to whether her conceptualisation of the education and training of nurses was underpinned by an equally zealous religious pragmatism.

III: *Nightingale's Concept of Nursing Education*

Work

The persistent theme of Nightingale's concept of nursing was its sanitary approach to matters of health and disease (Nightingale, 1859b, 1882b and 1893). As well as being inspired by her religious pragmatism, nursing as it ought to be done required 'knowledge, practice, self-abnegation, and ... direct obedience to, and activity under, the highest of all Masters, and from the highest of all motives' (Nightingale, 1865, pp. 10–11). Furthermore, Nightingale strongly believed that 'Man has the power to realize all that is right and good, not by prayers to another Being to do his work, not by a mysterious 'self determining' power through which he shall 'will' to do it, but by taking God's appointed means' (Nightingale, 1860a, p. 172), or as she once put it in a letter to Jowett summarised by Smith (Smith, 1982, p. 184):

> 'It is a religious act to clean out a gutter and to prevent cholera, and ... it is not a religious act to pray (in the sense of asking).' Moreover, she was divinely appointed to know. ... She reminded Jowett that ... she was uniquely 'part of God's plan. God had created her like Himself, "a Trainer", in a world which was "a training school."' Her task was to declare God's laws of sanitation and virtue, and to aid and measure each person's adherence to those laws and thereby guide the world's slow march towards perfection.

It is on the basis of such remarks that her religious pragmatism can be expected to have influenced her concept of nursing education.

Education

Learning

As shown earlier, Nightingale's concept of nursing was based upon her belief that the techniques of sanitary science, such as statistics, were given to man by God in order to enable him to discover his laws, his will. Next, it was up to man's free choice to bring his will in accordance with God's will (Nightingale, 1860b, pp. 53–54):

> *Man has capability to learn how circumstances regulate and modify human nature, to learn what circumstances develop and exercise human nature aright. By the united efforts of mankind, in accordance with God's ever-present, ever-efficient law, to bring about such circumstances is man's work. The capability for this is man's power.*

Nursing, as Nightingale viewed it, was thus one of the areas, and a very important one, for man to employ his power to learn the 'how' and the 'what' of human nature in order to develop and exercise it effectively. To achieve this, however, he needed some sort of education (Nightingale, 1873a, p. 576):

> *The facts of what is more strictly called education, though sanitary facts are one of the most powerful means of educating mankind, show, if possible, still more strongly what here has been imperfectly expressed. ... viz. That education is to teach men not to know, but to do; that the true end of education is production, that the object of education is not orna-mentation, but production – (after man has learnt to produce, then let him ornament himself) – but 'production' in the widest sense of the term. And, to teach man to produce, the educating him to perfect accuracy of thought – and, it might have been added, to accurate habits of observation – and to perfectly accurate habits of expression, is the main, the constant way – what a grand 'lesson' this is.*

This line of reasoning in one of Nightingale's writings on religion, if compared with her remarks on the training of nurses, is yet another proof of her consistency. To grasp its significance, however, one first has to note the parallelism with the requisites for Nightingale's religious concept of education:

- 'to learn how circumstances regulate and modify human nature' is on a par with 'accurate habits of observation',
- 'to learn what circumstances develop and exercise human nature aright' is on a par with 'perfect accuracy of thought',
- 'to bring about such circumstances' is on a par with 'accurate habits of expression.'

This was also the line of reasoning used by her in 'Nurses, training of' (Nightingale, 1882a, p. 321):

Observation tells how the patient is; reflection tells what is to be done; training tells how it is to be done. Training and experience are, of course, necessary to teach us, too, how to observe, what to observe; how to think, what to think. Observation tells us the fact; reflection the meaning of the fact. Reflection needs training as much as observation.

In order to grasp Nightingale's concept of nursing education, it seems appropriate to dwell upon Nightingale's views on observation, reflection and training. From the analysis of these views, it will become clear that Nightingale's writings on nursing education can be interpreted narrowly as well as broadly, and that it is the latter interpretation which provides a richer insight into her concept of nursing education.

Observation
'Notes on nursing' contains one chapter, entitled 'Observation of the sick', which is full of anecdotal examples of observation by nurses. These examples, however, are used to teach the following lesson (Nightingale, 1859b, p. 59):

The most important practical lesson that can be given to nurses is to teach them what to observe – how to observe – what symptoms indicate improvement – what the reverse – which are of importance – which are of none – which are the evidence of neglect – and of what kind of neglect.

On the next page, this skill of observation is contrasted with (1859b, p. 60, footnote), 'observation simple' in which, despite the exposure to sensory phenomena, nothing is observed, as well as 'observation compound, compounded, that is, with the imaginative faculty.' Whereas the information of the former was simply 'defective', that of the latter was 'much more dangerous' as it was based upon mere imagination. Nightingale thought the skill of observation to be so crucial that she advised mothers of families that 'if you cannot get the habit of observation one way or another, you had better give up the being a nurse, for it is not your calling, however kind and anxious you may be' (1859b, p. 63).

Two important aspects of observation she further pointed out were that the nurse must 'distinguish between the idiosyncracies of patients' (1859b, p. 66) and that observation also implied 'an inquiry into all the conditions in which the patient lives' (1859b, p. 68). Both aspects were of equal importance.

Although Nightingale held the view that man's behaviour was determined by the uniform relations between his condition and the circumstances affecting it, she did not fail to acknowledge certain idiosyncracies in human behaviour as well. These idiosyncracies she attributed to the fact that, up to a certain degree, some of the circumstances affecting the human condition were in each case unique and were never to be repeated again. As for the physical nature of man, this should be taken to mean that (Nightingale, 1860a, p. 12):

...certain conditions are essential to human life, others to the healthy existence of a human being; while, in other particulars, individuals vary as to those which are essential or conducive to health. But uniform relation is observable in all states in which human nature exists.

In 'Nurses, training of', Nightingale, partly repeating herself, elaborated on the subject of observation (Nightingale, 1882a, pp. 320–321):

The trained power of attending to one's own impressions made by one's own senses, so that these should tell the nurse how the patient is, is the sine quâ non of being a nurse at all. ... To look is not always to see. ... Without a trained power of observation, no nurse can be of any use in reporting to the medical attendant ... Neither can the nurse obey intelligently his directions. It is most important to observe the symptoms of illness; it is, if possible, more important still to observe the symptoms of nursing; of what is at fault not of the illness, but of the nursing.

These remarks highlighted, once again, that nursing proper was different from medicine, as the nurse's observation had to focus not only on the symptoms of illness but also on the uniform relations between the patient and the environmental circumstances affecting him. The nurse had thus to look for sanitary phenomena manifesting God's laws, and to that extent, nursing was an art to be performed independently from the physician or the surgeon, thereby placing it under the authority of God.

Reflection
Observation in itself was not enough as it had to be complemented by reflection, and this skill required training too (Nightingale, 1882a, p. 321):

Reflection needs training as much as observation. Otherwise the untrained nurse, like other people called quacks, easily falls into the confusion of 'on account of,' because 'after' – the blunder of the 'three crows'.

More than twenty years earlier, Nightingale had expressed the same concern in 'notes on nursing' (Nightingale, 1859b, p. 65):

Almost all superstitions are owing to bad observation, to the post hoc, ergo propter hoc; and bad observers are almost all superstitious. Farmers used to attribute disease among cattle to witchcraft; weddings have been

*attributed to seeing one magpie, deaths to seeing three; and I have heard
the most highly educated now-a-days draw consequences for the sick
closely resembling these.*

Clearly what Nightingale meant by reflection was the capacity of the
nurse to think about what she sees and for this thinking to influence her
actions. As she stated: 'Observation tells us the fact; reflection the
meaning of the fact.' It is interesting to note that Nightingale's injunction
at the end of the nineteenth century to think about what is being observed
and act on this is now – a century later – a central concept in the notion
of 'the reflective practitioner' being adopted in nursing under the influence of writers such as Schön (1983; 1987). Indeed, Nightingale's sugges-
tion that 'Observation tells *how* the patient is; reflection tells *what* is to be
done; training tells *how* it is to be done' (Nightingale, 1882a, p. 321) could
be taken in itself as a formula for the training and the practice of nursing.
Nightingale's remarks on the need for reflection, and for observation for
that matter too, it is contended here, should be interpreted against the
background of her positive theology in which she repeatedly pointed to
the dangers of:

- *thinking without observation*, which was on a par with superstitions
  as a result of the miraculous and the supernatural theology,
- *observation without thinking*, which was on a par with positivism.

Whereas positivists, notably Huxley, used to attack all sorts of theology
for being 'extra-belief (Aberglaube), meaning, not superstition, but belief
in things not verified by the senses', Nightingale herself accused Huxley
of advocating or succumbing to 'a sort of infra-belief; covering, indeed,
but small part of the ground man stands upon, less still of the horizon he
looks on' (Nightingale, 1873a, p. 568).

This broadened interpretation of Nightingale's remarks on the nurse's
observation and reflection is borne out by the way she discussed the third
requisite of nursing: training.

Training
Both in 'Nurses, training of' and in 'Sick nursing and health nursing',
Nightingale addressed the subject of training in two different ways. On
the one hand, she discussed training in a rather simple and straightfor-
ward manner (Nightingale, 1882a, p. 320):

*Training is to teach not only what is to be done, but how to do it. The
physician or surgeon orders what is to be done. Training has to teach the
nurse how to do it to his order; and to teach, not only how to do it, but*

why such and such a thing is done, and not such and such another; as also to teach symptoms, and what symptoms indicate what of disease or change, and the "reason why" of such symptoms.

On the other hand, Nightingale also discussed training in a wider sense (Nightingale, 1882a, p. 322):

To obey is to understand orders, and to understand orders really is to obey. A nurse does not know how to do what she is told without such "training" as enables her to understand what she is told; or without such moral and disciplinary "training" as enables her to give her whole self to obey.

This broadened meaning of training fitted in with her description of man's relationship to God –. 'the relation between a perfect creator, creating and training His creatures to perfection' (Nightingale, 1860a, p. 22). As for this relationship, man was not expected to obey blindly. On the contrary, he was expected to develop and exercise his God-given capabilities so as to enable him to bring his will in accordance with God's will. Not surprisingly, Nightingale advocated (Nightingale, 1860b, p. 246):

the substitution for authority ... of sense of truth and right, of accordance with right, adding that 'No longer can it be duty submitted to, but right accorded with, which must be the spirit of mankind. ... Truth, in our relations both with God and with man, must come in this substitution of accordance of the whole nature with right for authority, vaguely acknowledged from fear or duty.

Furthermore, this training in the wider sense also reflected on training in the narrow sense insofar as Nightingale held the opinion that:

Training has to make her [the nurse] not servile, but loyal to medical orders and authorities (Nightingale, 1882a, p. 333).

The opposite of this 'accordance with right' expected from the nurse was 'might is right.' The broader and above all moral interpretation of Nightingale's concept of training is borne out by her twofold definition of the nurse's training (Nightingale, 1893, p. 26; see also Nightingale, 1882a, pp. 333–334).

- *Training in the narrow sense* 'Training is to teach the nurse to help the patient to live. Nursing the sick is an art, and an art requiring an organized, practical and scientific training; for nursing is the skilled servant of medicine, surgery and hygiene. A good nurse of twenty years ago had not to do the twentieth part of what she is required by her physician or surgeon to do now; and so, after the year's training, she must be still training under instruction in her first and even second year's hospital service. The physician prescribes for supplying the vital force, but the nurse supplies it.'

- *Training in the wide sense* 'Training is to teach the nurse how God makes health, and how He makes disease. Training is to teach the nurse to know her business, that is, to observe exactly in such stupendous issues as life and death, health and disease. Training has to make her, not servile, but loyal to medical orders and authorities. True loyalty to orders cannot be without the independent sense or energy of responsibility, which alone secures real trustworthiness. Training is to teach the nurse to handle the agencies within our control which restore health and life, in strict, intelligent obedience to the physician's or surgeon's power and knowledge; how to keep the health mechanism prescribed to her in gear. Training must show her how the effects on life of nursing may be calculated with nice precision, such care or carelessness, such a sick rate, such duration of case, such a death-rate.'

Finally, whereas the former concept of training is related to the concept of nursing being ancillary to medicine, the latter concept corresponds most closely to Nightingale's concept of sanitary nursing and, by implication, to the service to God through the service to mankind.

Discipline: the essence of training

Nightingale's concept of training in the wide sense was a corollary of her concept of nursing. Underlying both these concepts was her religious pragmatism putting great emphasis upon statistical observation of sanitary phenomena, followed up by religious reflection and resulting in training and experience with regard to social reform.

The essence of Nightingale's concept of training was therefore of a moral and religious rather than an educational nature. This conclusion is corroborated by her concept of discipline emerging from it (Nightingale, 1882a, p. 334; see also Nightingale, 1893, p. 27):

And <u>discipline</u>— is the essence of training. People connect discipline with the idea of drill, standing at attention – some with flagellating themselves, some with flagellating boys. A lady who has, perhaps, more experience in training than anyone else, says: 'It is education, instruction, training – all that in fact goes to the full development of our faculties, moral, physical, and spiritual, not only for this life, but looking on this life as the training-ground for the future and higher life. Then discipline embraces order, method, and, as we gain some knowledge of the laws of nature ('God's *laws'), we not only see order, method, a place for everything, each its own work, but we find no waste of material or force or space; we find, too, no hurry; and we learn to have patience with our circumstances and ourselves; and so, as we go on learning, we become more disciplined, more content to work where we are placed, more anxious to fill our appointed work than to see the result thereof; and so God, no doubt, gives us the required patience and steadfastness to continue in our 'blessed drudgery,' which is the discipline He sees best for most of us.*

Nightingale's concept of education therefore amounted to a permanent and cyclical process of learning by means of observation, reflection and training, which, except for its religious connotations, was similar to Dewey's philosophy of education (see, for example, Dewey, 1938).

Conclusion

The analysis of Nightingale's original works has shown her concept of nursing education undoubtedly to have been influenced, not to say determined, by her religious pragmatism. This should not, however, be taken to mean that Nightingale succeeded in putting her concept of nursing education into practice in the first Nightingale training schools for nurses. This project went astray for two main reasons. One has to do with the reluctance on the part of the governors of St. Thomas's Hospital in London to accept a training school for nurses, but (Baly, 1986, p. 17):

If they were going to accept a cuckoo in the nest, a cuckoo other hospitals had refused, they were going to make sure that the nurses were under their control.

As a result the first two decades of the school were dominated by the battle between, on the one hand, the faction led by Mrs. Wardroper, the matron, who used the probationers as cheap pairs of hands, and, on the other, the Nightingale faction which defended the educational purposes of the school.

The other reason for the project's decline was the lack of a clearly articulated purpose for the school. Although, in 1872, a five-point plan was made to salvage the school, Nightingale omitted to outline the educational objectives as well as the theoretical content and the practical experiences needed to achieve these objectives. As a result (Prince, 1984, p. 160):

Nursing as a separate enterprise did not emerge. The failure to define the nursing job led not only to sisters and nurses not knowing what they should do, but not knowing what they should not do. The intellectual contribution to the curriculum was autonomously and capriciously decided by medical men; the practical experience, such as it was, by Matron and ward sisters.

At the end of the day, the Nightingale faction lost the battle. But, in spite of that, Nightingale kept in touch with the schools by means of the addresses to her nurses in which 'through the simple and popular style of the addresses something of a philosophical framework can be seen. When Miss Nightingale hopes that her nurses are a step further on the way to becoming 'perfect as our Father in Heaven is perfect,' she has in mind the conception she had formed of a moral government of the world in which science, activity, and religion were one' (Nash, 1914, p. vii).

IV: *Nightingale's concept of professional nursing*

Calling or profession

One of the issues to be addressed in every analysis of Nightingale's influence on the development of modern nursing is her stance on the question of whether nursing is a profession or not. Given the results of the analysis so far, it will come as no surprise that she thought nursing to be a calling rather than a profession, and this, too, was one of the persistent themes in her writings on nursing.

In these writings the theme of nursing being a calling emerged for the first time in 'Notes on nursing', when she wrote that it was better for mothers of families unable to master the skill of observation to give up being nurses, for it was not their calling.

This was long before the issue of whether nursing was a profession in its own right could even have been raised, as the nursing profession was nonexistent at the time. Nightingale's remarks on this issue in 'Notes on nursing' should, therefore, be interpreted within the context of her religious pragmatism rather than in relation to the controversy of 'calling versus profession.'

In 1893, however, when Nightingale wrote 'Sick nursing and health nursing', the situation had changed dramatically. Nursing was emerging as one of the new professions. Since 1886, the so-called 'Nurses Battle' over the State Registration for nurses was raging in Great Britain. In the United States, the campaign for professional recognition was being pursued more vigorously and, perhaps paradoxically, drew on Nightingale's work for its inspiration and justification. Although Nightingale still viewed nursing as a calling, her unchanged position contrasted sharply with the signs of the time.

Nursing: A calling from God

The best way of accounting for the position taken by Nightingale in 1859 is provided by her summary of 'Notes on nursing' which started with the following remarks (Nightingale, 1859b, p. 73):

> .. the answer to two of the commonest objections urged, one by women themselves, the other by men, against the desirableness of sanitary knowledge for women, plus a caution, comprises the whole argument for the art of nursing.

The way in which Nightingale elaborated on both these objections and the caution are most illuminating as to what she meant by nursing being a calling, because it shows that her position on this issue was also inspired by her religious pragmatism.

The first objection, put forward by men, drew attention to the danger of amateur 'physicking' by women as a result of teaching them the laws of health. To this Nightingale answered (Nightingale, 1859b, pp. 73–74):

> But this is just what the really experienced and observing nurse does not do; she neither physics herself nor others. And to cultivate in things pertaining to health observation and experience in women who are mothers, governesses or nurses, is just the way to do away with amateur physicking, and if the doctors did but know it, to make nurses obedient to them, – helps to them instead of hindrances. Such education in women would indeed diminish the doctor's work – but no one really believes that doctors wish that there should be more illness, in order to have more work.

Both this objection and Nightingale's reaction to it were concerned with the need to teach women the skills of health observation and experience, not in terms of amateur 'physicking' which had to do with disease but as the conditio sine qua non for promoting health. This was, however (as shown earlier) only the first stage in the development of nursing and it inevitably gave rise to heightened public interest in the laws of health.

The second objection, put forward by women themselves, was that they could not know anything of the laws of health because they could know nothing of pathology and could not dissect. To this 'confusion of ideas which it is hard to attempt to dissentangle' Nightingale answered by comparing the lessons to be learnt from pathology, on the one hand, and observation and experience, on the other (1859b, p. 74):

> Pathology teaches the harm that disease has done. But it teaches nothing more. We know nothing of the principle of health, the positive of which

pathology is the negative, except from observation and experience. And nothing but observation and experience will teach us the ways to maintain or to bring back the state of health. It is often thought that medicine is the curative process. It is no such thing; medicine is the surgery of functions, as surgery proper is that of limbs and organs. Neither can do anything but remove obstructions; neither can cure; nature alone cures. ... And what nursing has to do in either case, is to put the patient in the best condition for nature to act upon him.

This objection, and Nightingale's reaction to it, were concerned with observation and experience as the subject matter for reflection, or with the question of what lesson was to be learnt. In Nightingale's opinion, the positive lesson taught by observation and experience, i.e. the principle of health, was far more valuable than the negative lesson taught by pathology, i.e. the harm the disease had done.

She furthermore emphasised that it was not medicine but nature that cured, and it was nursing rather than medicine or surgery which had to help nature by putting the patient in the best condition for nature to act upon him. By adding this information, and not for the first time, Nightingale changed the tone of the argument from purely scientific to religious: health observation and experience existed to teach man not only the principle of health but also the laws of nature which constituted the laws of God, resulting in a process of learning by experience and careful inquiry.

The caution which ended Nightingale's summary of 'Notes on nursing' was directed against (Nightingale, 1859b, p. 75):

the commonly received idea among men and even among women themselves that it requires nothing but a disappointment in love, the want of an object, a general disgust, or incapacity for other things, to turn a woman into a good nurse.

This should not be taken to mean that Nightingale favoured the idea of nursing as a profession, as opposed to the romanticised idea of nursing as a calling. On the contrary, she argued (Nightingale, 1859b, p. 75):

... the knowing what are the laws of life and death for men, and what the laws of health for wards ... are not these matters of sufficient importance and difficulty to require learning by experience and careful inquiry, just as much as any other art? They do not come by inspiration to the lady disappointed in love, nor to the poor workhouse drudge hard up for a livelihood.

In other words, sanitary nursing, as Nightingale wanted mothers of families to practise it, required a positive commitment to learning the laws of life and death, i.e. the laws of God, and acting accordingly. This religious interpretation is prompted by Nightingale's comparison of the commitment demanded from Roman Catholic nurses and that of the English mothers of families: 'It is true we make no "vows." But is a "vow" necessary to convince us that the true spirit for learning any art, most specially an art of charity, aright, is not a disgust to everything or something else? Do we really place the love of our kind (and of nursing, as one branch of it) so low as this?' (Nightingale 1859b, pp. 75–76).

Nightingale's summarisation of 'Notes on nursing' portrayed the art of nursing as an instance of man's relationship with God, involving both a calling from God and efforts on the part of the nurse to make her election sure (see also Nightingale, 1893, p. 32). Outlining her position, however, she also mentioned the value of nursing and medicine and the role of men and women in society. Both these elements may give rise to an interpretation of Nightingale's position different from the one put forward here.

Nightingale viewed nursing as a calling rather than a profession which followed the footsteps of the medical profession. In 'Suggestions for thought' Nightingale has articulated her view of a profession, (Nightingale, 1860b, p. 5, footnote):

> a set of men paid to *profess* some kind of opinions; the clergy are paid to profess one kind of religion, the Wesleyans another. In the medical profession, the allopath is paid to profess one system of medicine, the homoeopath another. And all have their small families to support.

This description is not only consistent with Nightingale's judgment of opinions on the basis of the good they created for mankind rather than by the income they generated, but it also explains the manifold references to the differences between nursing and medicine in her writings, aimed at emphasising the moral implications of nursing which were conspicuously absent in medicine.

Nightingale's description of a profession also suggests that, whereas medicine was men's work, nursing was women's work. This interpretation is vindicated by Nightingale's statement that nursing was an activity for which women were gifted with a special aptitude (Nightingale, 1859a, p. 54):

> ... the woman is superior in skill to the man in all points of sanitary domestic economy, and more particularly in cleanliness and tidiness.

Great sanitary civil reformers will always tell us that they look to the woman to carry out practically their hygienic reforms. She has a superior aptitude in <u>nursing</u> the well quite as much as in nursing the sick.

In the book from which this quotation is taken, 'Notes on hospitals', Nightingale also compared 'personal hygiene' with 'public hygiene' (Nightingale, 1859a, pp. 46–47). Similar to the physician or the surgeon who was in charge of the hygiene of his patients, she argued, the army had to have at its disposal an officer of health in charge of the hygiene of buildings, to which it can be added that, whereas the former dealt with disease, the latter was concerned with health. It remains to be seen, however, whether these two roles were sex-linked or not.

Nightingale's summary of 'Notes on nursing' contains too many references to the opinions of men and women to be simply ignored. The main question is whether the texts analysed here should be interpreted within a feminist perspective (Smith, 1981) or not.

Admittedly, the second volume of 'Suggestions for thought' contains, apart from the text of 'Cassandra' (Nightingale, 1860b, pp. 374–411) which some consider to be one of the classics in feminist literature (Poovey, 1991), many autobiographical references to the position of girls and women in Victorian society. Perhaps these references reflect Nightingale's own conflicts, especially with her mother and her sister. They leave us in doubt as to the degree to which Nightingale's life had been affected by her family disagreeing with what she did. On the other hand, her Unitarian beliefs, which favoured a more active role for women in occupations, may have played a role as well.

However, in contrast with many of Nightingale's remarks on the position of women in Victorian society, it definitely was not her intention to present nursing as a calling within the context of the feminist cause for women's rights, for at the end of her summary of 'Notes on nursing', she added a footnote (Nightingale, 1859b, p. 75) in which she asked her 'sisters to keep clear ... of the jargon ... about the "rights" of women, which urges women to do all that men do, including the medical and other professions, merely because men do it, and without regard to whether this is the best that women can do.' This was not to say that they should not keep clear of other jargon, namely 'the jargon which urges women to do nothing that men do, merely because they are women, and should be "recalled to a sense of duty as women." and because "this is women's work," and "that is men's," and "these are things which women should not do," which is all assertion and nothing more.' It was typical of

Nightingale that her religious belief transcended both these positions (Nightingale, 1859b, p. 75):

> Surely woman should bring the best she has, _whatever_ that is, to the work of God's world, without attending to either of these cries. ... Oh, leave these jargons, and go your way straight to God's work, in simplicity and singleness of heart.

Nightingale's religiously inspired position on the issue of nursing being a calling was probably prompted by her conviction that, on at least four occasions (1837, 1853, 1854, and 1861), she was 'called' by God to do the work she did. In addition, the position taken by her also reflected her religious pragmatism leading to its logical conclusion, for, granted that man was afforded the inducements as well as the means to advance in the knowledge, will and power needed to approximate the union with God, it would be a folly to exclude women from both the inducements and the means to participate in mankind's serving God through serving mankind. This was a position probably few modern feminists would be willing to subscribe to.

A progressive calling

In 'Nursing the sick', written some two decades after the publication of 'Notes on nursing', Nightingale did not explicitly state that she saw nursing as a calling, except at the end of the article. There she characterised nursing as a progressive calling, pointing to the fact that (Nightingale, 1882b, p. 349):

> Year by year nurses have to learn new and improved methods, as medicine and surgery and hygiene improve. Year by year nurses are called upon to do more and better than they have done. It is felt to be impossible to have a public register of nurses that is not a delusion. ... Further, year by year, nursing needs to be more and more of a moral calling.

As she had written 'Nursing the sick' as an entry for a medical dictionary, Nightingale probably had to abstain from mentioning religious beliefs underlying her concept of nursing and nursing education too explicitly. Nevertheless, as has been shown from her remarks on the training of nurses (Nightingale, 1882a, pp. 333–334), she managed to put in enough religious content to be seen not to have changed her mind at all.

This explains why, at first sight, Nightingale's rejection of a public register appeared to be founded upon the continuous innovation and improvement of the methods of nursing as a result of advances in medicine, surgery and hygiene. Having made her point in this generally acceptable way, she superimposed the actual reason, which was that the moral dimension of nursing was incompatible with such a public register. This interpretation of Nightingale's position is vindicated by her descriptions of what she considered to be a good nurse (see Table 3).

Assuming that this interpretation is correct, it once again confirms Nightingale's consistency, this time with regard to the issue of nursing being a calling rather than a profession. Her opposition to a public register of nurses was based not so much upon scientific developments as upon her belief that nursing was a progressive process of learning about the laws of God.

In the light of Nightingale's religious pragmatism, her remarks therefore should be taken to mean that nursing was a calling for two reasons. Firstly, as a result of medicine, surgery and hygiene improving year by year, nurses were increasingly able to learn the laws of nature with regard to man's physical mode of being. Secondly, as a result of applying these laws of nature nurses became part of God's plan, that man would bring his own will in accordance with God's will. This religious outlook on the nature of nursing she never abandoned.

Calling versus profession
It is beyond doubt that Nightingale viewed nursing as a calling from as early as the 1850s and possibly even earlier than that. Nothing, not even the emergence of the profession of nursing, could bring her to change her position on this issue. This assessment of her position is vindicated by the way in which she expressed her hopes for the future of nursing as late as 1893 (Nightingale, 1893, pp. 36–37):

> *May we hope that the nurse may understand more and more of the moral and material government of the world by the Supreme Moral Governor – higher, better, holier, than her 'own acts,' that government which enwraps her round, and by which her own acts must be led, with which her own acts must agree in their due proportion, in order that this, the highest hope of all, may be hers; raising her above, i.e., putting beneath her, dangers, fashions, mere money-getting, solitary money-getting, but availing herself of the high helps that may be given her by the sympathy and support of good 'homes'; raising her above intrusive personal mortifications, pride in her own proficiency (she may have a just pride in her own doctors and training-school), sham, and clap-trap; raising her to the highest 'grade' of all – to be a fellow-worker with the Supreme Good, with God! That she may be a 'graduate' in this, how high! that she may be a 'graduate' in words, not realities, how low! We are only on the threshold of nursing.*

Table 3 Nightingale's image of the nurse (Nightingale, 1882b, p. 351).

A really good nurse must needs be of the highest class of character. It need hardly be said that she must be -

(1) Chaste, in the sense of the Sermon on the Mount; a good nurse should be the Sermon on the Mount in herself. ...

(2) Sober, in spirit as well as in drink, and temperate in all things.

(3) Honest, not accepting the most trifling fee or bribe from patients or friends.

(4) Truthful - and to be able to tell the truth includes attention and observation, to observe truly - memory, to remember truly - power of expression, to tell truly what one has observed truly - as well as intention to speak the truth, the whole truth, and nothing but the truth.

(5) Trustworthy, to carry out directions intelligently and perfectly, unseen as well as seen, "to the Lord" as well as unto men - no mere eye-service.

(6) Punctual to a second, and orderly to a hair ...

(7) Quiet, yet quick; quick without a hurry; gentle without slowness; discreet without self-importance; no gossip.

(8) Cheerful, hopeful; not allowing herself to be discouraged by unfavourable symptoms; not given to depress the patient by anticipations of an unfavourable result.

(9) Cleanly to the point of exquisiteness, both for the patient's sake and her own; neat and ready.

(10) Thinking of her patient and not of herself; "tender over his occasions" or wants, cheerful and kindly, patient, ingenious and *feat*. The best definition can be found, as always, in Shakespeare, where he says that to be "nurse-like" is to be

> *'So kind, so duteous, diligent,*
> *So tender over his occasions, true,*
> *So feat.'*

This was the very same position taken by Nightingale in 1859 (in 'Notes on nursing') and 1882 (in 'Nursing the sick'), except for its changed context, namely the debate between nursing as a calling and nursing as a profession. Nightingale's hopes for the future of nursing, and especially her remark on the threshold of nursing, were somehow paralleled by God's vision of man entering the kingdom of heaven (Nightingale, 1860b, p. 205):

> *The 'kingdom of heaven is within,' indeed, but it must also create one without, because we are <u>intended</u> to act upon our circumstances. We must*

beware, both of thinking that we can maintain that 'kingdom of heaven within' under all circumstances, – because there are circumstances under which the human being cannot be good, and also of thinking that the kingdom of heaven <u>without</u> will produce that <u>within</u>.

Moreover, Nightingale's view of nursing being a calling from God rather than a profession adds a religious significance to the dangers she summed up in this last authoritative statement on nursing matters (Nightingale, 1893, pp. 34):

To sum up the dangers:

1. *On one side, fashion, and want of earnestness, not making it a life but a mere interest consequent on this;*
2. *On the other side, mere money-getting; yet man does not live by bread alone, still less women.*
3. *Making it a profession, and no calling. Not making your 'calling and election sure,' wanting especially with private nurses, the community of feeling of a common nursing home, pressing towards the 'mark of your high calling,' keeping up the moral tone.*
4. *Above all, danger of making it book-learning and lectures – not an apprenticeship, a workshop practice.*
5. *Thinking that any hospital with a certain number of beds may be a box to train nurses in, regardless of the conditions essential to a sound hospital organization, especially the responsibility of the female head for the conduct and discipline of the nurses.*
6. *Imminent danger of stereotyping instead of progressing. 'No system can endure that does not march.' Objects of registration not capable of being gained by a public register. Who is to guarantee our guarantors? Who is to make the inquiries? You might as well register mothers as nurses. A good nurse must be a good woman.*

One of these so-called dangers, namely state registration by means of a public register, was at the source of the long lasting conflict between Nightingale and the British Nurses Association led by Mrs. Bedford Fenwick. In a historical study of this conflict (Mills & Dale, 1964, p. 35), Nightingale is said to have been strongly opposed to the use of the word 'profession' in relation to nursing. Instead, she preferred the word 'calling', because she 'did not appear to have a very high opinion of her own sex, and was not disposed to help the progress of the emancipation of women.'

Both the reasons put forward by Mills and Dale (ibid.) are at variance with Nightingale's real position, which was based upon her religious pragmatism. In a letter of 1892, for example, she asked Miss March, one of her correspondents, 'to "pray for the nurses and nursing," for nursing had become "the fashion" with emphasis on registering and wages rather than on duty in the sense of "work for God" (summarised by Monteiro, 1972, p. 528).

All this goes a long way to show that, as far as Nightingale was concerned, nursing was not a profession in need of some religious justification. On the contrary, for her nursing was a religious activity based upon a calling from God which should not be compromised by such mundane interests as fashion, money-making, registration, emancipation of women and so on.

V: *The Application of Nightingale's Concept of Nursing*

Survival of the concept
The major problem to be faced in the search for applications of Nightingale's concept of nursing is the lack of an identifiable group of followers of Nightingale's sanitary approach to nursing, similar to, for example, the psychoanalysts following Freud's approach.

This is not to say that the sanitary measures advocated by her have failed to influence the practice of nursing. On the contrary, these measures have been very much in evidence in the textbooks of nursing written ever since.

But it is quite another thing to say that these textbooks were based on the principles of sanitary science, for they definitely were not. This observation is in sharp contrast with Levine's appraisal of the lasting significance of Nightingale's principles of nursing (Levine, 1963, p. 28):

> *So solid and basic were these principles that they never changed. For fifty years she espoused them, and not even the development of the germ theory could shake her conviction or, more remarkably, the esssential validity of her principles.*

Bishop (1960, p. 249), in a discussion about Nightingale's message for today, took this even further when he wrote that:

> *.. in regard to the fundamentals of nursing, I think it is true that Florence Nightingale's prevision was such that no first principle laid down by her has needed alteration, or is likely to.*

Both Levine's and Bishop's evaluation of the long-term significance of Nightingale's concept of nursing are somewhat misleading for, while many sanitary measures advocated by Nightingale were undoubtedly very effective and still make sense, the theory of miasmatism underlying such measures has become obsolete ever since the discoveries of bacteriology confirmed the contagionist point of view.

Other appraisals of Nightingale's concept of nursing which take into account the substitution of bacteriology for sanitary science come from Palmer (1977) and Baly (1969). Whereas the former (Palmer, 1977, p. 87) emphasised Nightingale's rejection of the germ theory as an example of her reactionary character, the latter (Baly, 1969, p. 2) reached a more positive conclusion:

'Notes on nursing' preceded the germ theory of infection, yet with an almost incredible perspicacity they foreshadow it. "Lack of health teaching" is the theme.

At least, this appraisal does some justice to one of Nightingale's lasting contributions to the development of nursing – the nurse in the role of the health-missioner, which was to result in the increasing acceptance of the public health nurse.

On the other hand, it glosses over the wider implications of the differences between miasmatism and contagionism which, in the final analysis, give rise to two contrasting approaches to nursing. It is this contrast which may explain why Nightingale's concept of nursing has failed to result in what could be rightly called a Nightingale school of nursing.

Miasmatism and contagionism revisited

The main reason why Nightingale's concept of nursing has not attracted a group of avowed followers, it is contended here, was her taking sides with the advocates of the theory of miasmatism as well as her subsequent rejection of the germ theory. The latter was not, however, the only implication of the position taken by her, for both miasmatism and contagionism have much wider implications, as both represent a more general orientation or conceptual framework. In his doctoral study on the relationships between medicine and philosophy, Ten Have (1983, pp. 229–316) has undertaken a detailed comparison of these explanatory theories of epidemic diseases from which most of the following analysis is drawn.

Miasmatism

According to the theory of miasmatism, epidemic diseases are caused by impurities in the environment of man. The exact nature of these impurities has given rise to much speculation. Whereas Hippocrates, the acclaimed originator of miasmatism, held air, water, soil, climate and the seasons to be responsible for most epidemic diseases, the miasmatists of the last century pointed to more specific circumstances of living like putrified water, lack of proper ventilation, garbage, excrements, rotten food, and so on, as the source of so-called miasmata (whatever these miasmata may have been, for their existence has never been demonstrated beyond any doubt).

Because of these miasmata, man was held to become increasingly susceptible to epidemic diseases which, according to the miasmatists, could not be transmitted from one individual to the other.

Ten Have (1983, pp. 233–235) summarises the miasmatic position by pointing to the following characteristics. According to the miasmatic explanation of the genesis of epidemic diseases, the environment was the active agent and the individual the passive recipient of miasmata. Further, medical treatment of epidemic disease was directed at manipulating the environmental causes rather than treating the individual affected by the disease, and, although the prevention of epidemic disease was held to be feasible by means of improving sanitation, separating healthy from diseased persons (quarantine) was not considered to be a useful measure. Not surprisingly, most miasmatists of the last century were also fervent supporters of social and political reform. A third characteristic of the miasmatic position was that everything was seen as interrelated and interdependent. As a result of this so-called universalistic attitude, intervention in one part was considered to be utterly useless unless other relevant factors were dealt with as well. Finally, at the source of these characteristics of the miasmatic approach was the multicausal and interdependent explanation of disease.

Contagionism
According to the theory of contagionism, originating from the Judaeo-Christian tradition, epidemic diseases are caused by small living entities called contagia. These contagia were believed to be able to enter the living body, to multiply themselves, to be eliminated and to be transmitted to another living body by means of bodily contact, by air and by clothes and other objects. To appreciate the discussion during the first half of the nineteenth century it is worth bearing in mind that, until the discovery of the germ theory during the 1860s, this contagionist explanation of epidemic diseases was no less fanciful than that of miasmatism.

In summarising the contagionist position, Ten Have (1983, pp. 233–235) points out that, whereas the individual in which the contagia multiplied themselves played the active role in the genesis of the disease, the environment being the medium of transmission was attributed the passive role. In contrast with the miasmatic approach, medical treatment of epidemic disease initially focused on the stringent separation or quarantine of all individuals affected by the disease from healthy individuals, thereby foreshadowing the later emphasis upon the individual's biological structure and functions as well as his psychological make-up. Also in contrast with the miasmatic approach, medical treatment was directed at the adjustment of the individual to his environment, which was held to be unchangeable and static. The conceptual framework of contagionism was characterised by an atomistic orientation, as it focused upon the individual or parts of the individual which were seen as separate elements to be analysed in isolation from each other and to be treated by means of mechanical manipulation. Finally, at the source of these characteristics of the contagionist approach was the relatively monocausal explanation of disease, 'relatively' because some held the contagia to be disease-specific while others did not.

Two different orientations

Ten Have's analysis of miasmatism and contagionism has effectively exposed two different orientations or conceptual frameworks in medicine (Ten Have, 1983, pp. 235–236):

> *Whereas the theory of contagionism represents medicine in its orientation towards man himself, the individual, or the processes within the organism: his structure, his functions and his identifiable diseases, miasmatism stands for the orientation towards the environmental variables, or the environment in the widest meaning of the word: society, the pattern of living, the circumstances of living, the culture as well as the water, the air and the soil.*

Ten Have describes the contagionism orientation as the 'biological approach', a name which reflects the meaning of the Greek word 'bios' in both its somatic and psychological connotations. However, to exclude any environmental orientation and to put even more emphasis upon the orientation towards the individual, he also suggests the use of adjectives like 'personal' and 'individual'. Ten Have himself, however, prefers the term 'biological' because this name also implies specific methods of studying and practising medicine, i.e. the methods of natural science.

As for the miasmatism orientation, Ten Have describes it as the 'sociological approach', or alternatively, the 'ecological approach'. Yet another alternative, one which he himself prefers but rejects because it is an English word (the study was written in Dutch), is the term 'environmentalism'. On the other hand, one of the advantages of naming it the 'sociological approach' is that it implies the use of specific methods of study too, viz. the methods of social science.

Modern medicine
Having established these two different orientations underlying the controversy between miasmatism and contagionism, Ten Have sets out to demonstrate the existence of both the sociological and the biological approach in modern medicine. For this, he uses conflicting views as to the cause and the treatment of psychiatric diseases, alcoholism, heroin addiction, cardiovascular diseases and cancer. Whereas, for example, traditional psychiatry is characterised by a somatic and individual orientation, the anti-psychiatry movement emphasises societal and social factors in the genesis and the treatment of psychiatric diseases.

Following a similar line of argument for the other examples, Ten Have concludes that the controversy between miasmatism and contagionism should be interpreted as an example of the ongoing debate between the sociological and biological approach which is also taking place in modern medicine as (Ten Have, 1983, p. 252):

> *On the one hand, there is the biological approach focusing on the individual organism, looking for the causes of disease in somatic and psychic disorders of the functions and structures of the individual and directing medical treatment at the physical and mental condition of the individual or his personal patterns of behavior. On the other hand, there is the sociological approach focused primarily on the environment of man, identifying the causes of disease in the physical or social environment, in the circumstances of living, nutrition, the political system, in short in factors external to the individual, while interventions are directed at influencing these supra-individual factors.*

Philosophy and science
Ten Have then widens the debate between the sociological and the biological approach in modern medicine to philosophy and science as well. Whereas, for example in philosophy, the sociological approach is associated with empiricism, the theory of the tabula rasa, sensualism, and critical rationalism, the biological approach is related to rationalism, the theory of innate ideas, intellectualism, and inductivism. A similar situation can be found in linguistics where structuralism is in contrast with transformational-generative grammar. In psychology the sociological approach is represented by associational psychology, functionalism and behaviourism, while neo-Freudianism, Gestalt-psychology and humanistic psychology represent the biological approach. In biology the oppos-

ing approaches come to the fore in the controversy between nurture (environment) and nature (heredity).

Given the existence of these contrasting approaches in philosophy and science, Ten Have then arrives at the conclusion that the controversy between miasmatism and contagionism does not stand on its own but should be viewed as an example of the debate between the sociological and the biological approach which exists not only in medicine but in philosophy and science as well. To this it should be added that Ten Have does not think of this debate as a dichotomy between two points of view in which one excludes the other. On the contrary, the development of medicine, philosophy and science shows the contrasting approaches to be complementary to each other to the effect that they alternatively dominate the developments in these fields.

Finally, Ten Have's conclusion that the differences between miasmatism and contagionism mirror the wider debate between the sociological and biological approach in medicine, philosophy and science, justifies the use of his results for assessing the practical bearings of Nightingale's concept of nursing.

Death of the concept?
As far as the practical bearings of Nightingale's concept of nursing are concerned, these correspond with the sociological rather than the biological approach.

Firstly, Nightingale considered man's physical and moral condition to be subject to the laws of nature, exemplified by the uniform ways in which the circumstances of living affected man's physical and moral mode of being. In her opinion, it was, therefore, the environment which played the active role, while man was the passive recipient of environmental influences.

Secondly, to change the condition of man for better or worse required the manipulation of the environmental circumstances affecting it, thereby effectively changing the uniform relations between the individual and his environment. Nursing, as Nightingale viewed it, amounted therefore to some sort of 'environmental engineering'. Indirectly, this interpretation is vindicated by her fierce opposition to quarantine, which she liked to ridicule for its many untenable regulations, and, directly, by her political efforts to bring about sanitary reform.

Thirdly, the individual came into play only insofar as he was the one who had to take the moral decision for or against improving the circumstances in which he lived. To guard against any dichotomy between the moral and physical condition of man, it is necessary to point out once again that Nightingale held both conditions to be subject to the laws of nature. They were, however, different insofar as man's bodily condition needed to be healthy in order to develop and exercise his moral condition aright. This interrelatedness and interdependence between the individual and his environment was paralleled by an interrelatedness and interdependence on a greater scale – God's wise and beneficent government of the world, which showed man to be in the hands of God. This parallelism, it is contended here, is not only similar to the classic idea of the microcosmos of man corresponding to the macrocosmos of the universe, but also exemplifies Nightingale's universalistic attitude.

Finally, at the source of Nightingale's position was her conviction that man's well-being depended not only upon the manipulation of circumstances affecting his physical mode of being (sanitation) but also upon his moral decision to adapt his own free will to the will of God. As a result of this position, Nightingale saw it as the nurse's task to help man to live by teaching him about both the inducement and the means for the manipulation of environmental factors affecting his physical condition. Thereby, she also helped him to live in a morally right way for, to the degree that man adapted his free will to the will of God, he became increasingly one with God too. This implication of her concept of nursing reflects her attitude to the multicausality and the interdependence involved in the practice of nursing.

Despite her religiously inspired references to some individualising aspects of nursing, Nightingale's concept of nursing exemplifies the selfsame characteristics of the sociological approach as have been identified by Ten Have (op. cit.). Given that, during the second half of the nineteenth century, nursing became ancillary to medicine in which the biological approach was becoming increasingly dominant, Nightingale's concept of nursing stood little chance of general acceptance within the nursing community. What nurses did follow, however, were the hygienic measures, advocated by Nightingale, which were evidently not incompatible with the emerging bacteriological explanation and treatment of disease. In other words, Nightingale's concept of nursing, unlike many of the hygienic measures proposed by her, can be said to have died with her, and probably at an even earlier date.

VI: *The Meaning of the Nightingale Model of Nursing*

The basis of the model

An important point to bear in mind is that Nightingale herself did not speak of nursing models, nor did she give her name to a model of nursing as such. The notion of nursing models has in effect only come to the fore in the last quarter of a century or so.

It is not the intention of this brief work to embark upon a detailed critique of the notion of models and how they relate to other entities, such as theories, conceptual frameworks or discipline paradigms. Generally speaking, a model is a representation of some other phenomenon which exists in reality (Kaplan, 1964). It may be a physical replica, closely resembling the original, usually produced to scale and sometimes even a fully 'working' model of the original. Conversely, it may represent the original phenomenon by symbols – words and/or mathematical signs – and as such bear no physical resemblence to the original. A *conceptual* model is one in which the words or phrases which represent the parts of the original phenomenon are *concepts* i.e. abstract linkages of ideas such as man, person, table, pain. The model shows the concepts and how they are linked and interrelated: a conceptual model is therefore a framework for understanding reality.

A *nursing model* is therefore a conceptual model, constructed for the specific purposes of conceptualising the phenomenon of nursing. Because it is a broad and fairly abstract framework, some (such as Fawcett, 1993) see a nursing model as quite different from a nursing theory, which is said to be less abstract and more precise in describing causal relationships between concepts and the predictability of such relationships. Others (such as Chinn and Kramer, 1991) point to the tendency among nursing authors to be less than clear about any difference between nursing theories and nursing models. They elect instead to see models and theories as being largely synonymous and (as suggested by Meleis, 1991) argue that the business of attempting to differentiate between them is largely an exercise in semantics which takes away from the serious study of nursing.

In the context discussed here, a model of nursing is taken to be a broad conceptualisation of nursing. Although Florence Nightingale did not *explicitly* propose such a model, a framework of linked and interrelated concepts which outline her explication of nursing and which underpin her views on nursing education and professional nursing is indeed *implicit* in her writings. It is this *Nightingale model*, implicit in her writings, which is discussed here.

The analysis of the Nightingale model of nursing, put forward here, arises from Nightingale being characterised as a 'passionate statistician'. Underlying her model of nursing was the religious belief that the laws of nature manifested God's laws which man had to find out by the use of statistics. The major area in which she used this approach was sanitation. Nightingale's religious beliefs originated from her dissatisfaction with the teachings of the Christian churches which, in her opinion, amounted to mere reflection without observation, and the philosophy of positivism which she considered to result in mere observation without reflection. By combining observation (statistics) and reflection (religion), she developed her so-called positive theology which, at the end of the day, had to result in some sort of social (i.e. sanitary) reform.

Religion, as Nightingale saw it, was therefore something neither to be affirmed, for example by praying to God or by confirming the articles of faith, nor to be denied by excluding the possibility of man having any knowledge of God. On the contrary, religion required a moral commitment: it had to be lived and to be practised, for, using his intelligence to discover God's laws and his free will to adapt his behaviour to these laws, man was capable of working out his own happiness and advancing towards perfection. That, she strongly believed, was the way in which God had envisaged man learning about His character.

Further, it was Cook's (1913a) pointing to the similarities between Nightingale's positive theology and the pragmatist philosophy of his time that gave rise to the subsequent analysis of Nightingale's writings on nursing against the background of her religious pragmatism. This analysis has resulted in a reappraisal of the Nightingale model of nursing which, in many respects, is at variance with other interpretations.

Nightingale's religious pragmatism, this highly idiosyncratic mixture of science and theology and its accessory empirical and speculative methods, which was to result in social reform, provided her with an approach which showed up time and again in her writings on nursing and was characterised by the combination of observation, reflection, training and experience. Another feature which emerged from Nightingale's writings on nursing was her approach to nursing which was characterised by what Ten Have (op. cit.) called the sociological or environmentalist approach, as opposed to the biological approach.

Obviously, to grasp the full meaning of the Nightingale model of nursing one has to take into account her religious presuppositions as well as her sociological approach to nursing. Yet another way of interpreting this model of nursing is by taking Nightingale's writings at face value and using them to suit one's purposes. Both approaches will be discussed in more detail in the following summarisation of Nightingale's concepts of nursing, nursing education and the nursing profession.

The paradigm of nursing
It is generally suggested that, at any particular time, a discipline is guided by particular shared concepts and theoretical perspectives, concerns itself with common issues or problems, and adopts its own particular methods for addressing these issues. The term *paradigm* has been used to describe such a perspective (see, for example, Kuhn, 1970).

When the areas of concern are presented in their most fundamental form, beyond which further reduction is not possible, this is spoken of as the discipline's metaparadigm. A metaparadigm, is in fact the most abstract reduction of a discipline to its essential elements. Fawcett (1984; 1989) presented what is perhaps the most commonly referred-to metaparadigm of nursing, in which she identifies the discipline's major areas of concern as

- person
- environment
- health
- nursing

For a nursing model to be a true conceptual model of nursing, it is argued, it must address in a comprehensive way all the elements in the metaparadigm. It would appear that the Nightingale model does, to a greater or lesser extent, address the four metaparadigmatic elements proposed by Fawcett. The strengths and weaknesses of the model can therefore be analysed within this framework, as illustrated here.

Person

Generally speaking, the person emerging from Nightingale's writings on nursing is a rather passive one, susceptible as he is held to be to the range of circumstances affecting his different modes of being. This interpretation seems to be vindicated by Nightingale's admonition that 'Half the battle of nursing is to relieve your sick from having to think for themselves at all – least of all for their own nursing' (Nightingale, 1882b, p. 352), thereby implying that it was the nurse rather than the patient who was in charge of manipulating the circumstances affecting his health.

The passivity implied by man's condition being subject to factors external to him, however, is in contrast with the person's allegedly free will which enabled him to decide for or against changing these circumstances. It is on the basis of this free will that Welch (1986) set out to reconstruct Nightingale's views on the person and arrived at the conclusion that (Welch, 1986, p. 9):

> Her concept of the person is multidimensional and includes the following characteristics: (1) goal of life is oneness with God and nature, (2) knowledge of God's laws gives one power over the environment, (3) happiness is dependent upon one's knowledge and capabilities, (4) freedom and free will are gained through knowledge of God's laws, (5) one utilizes one's senses, direct observation, and experience to gain knowledge, and (6) one's knowledge of truth releases one from blind acceptance of authority. This person is much more active, dynamic, and creative than the one described in the role of the patient in Notes on Nursing.

Welch's conclusion therefore raises the question of whether Nightingale's views on the person implied either passivity or activity, or both, on the part of the individual.

The discussion about the relationship between necessity and free will, as Nightingale viewed it, has shown that, in the final analysis, her line of reasoning was bound to end up in deadlock because of the circular reasoning it was based upon. She tried to avoid this deadlock by resorting to the fact that man has to learn by experience.

The feasibility of this solution rested upon the assumption that man's different modes of being were related to each other by means of uniform relations of succession. This element of succession created an interval between one mode of being and the other, thereby giving man enough time for observation and reflection to change his behaviour accordingly. Because of this element of succession the rules of formal logic did not come into it any more. To illustrate this effect, one only has to look at the following propositions:

a. she married (p) and became pregnant (q),
b. she became pregnant (q) and married (p).

As far as formal logic is concerned, both these propositions have exactly the same meaning:

$$p + q = q + p.$$

In most people's experience, however, these propositions have quite different meanings. The explanation for this discrepancy between formal logic and human experience is the element of time which logic is incapable of dealing with, on the one hand, but which enables man to draw practical lessons from his experience through time, on the other hand. This was Nightingale's solution for the deadlock between necessity and free will.

This should not be taken to mean that every individual had to go through this process of learning by experience himself. On the contrary, it was mankind as a whole rather than each individual person who had to do this. Furthermore, this process of learning by mankind was dependent upon the emergence of so-called 'saviours' from either physical or moral errors. What Newton, for example, had been with regard to the former, Nightingale thought herself to be in relation to the latter. These saviours were supposed to actively discover the laws of God, while others had to do nothing but absorb and apply the lessons contained in these laws.

Finally, Welch's attempt to reconstruct Nightingale's views on the person was bound to fail, as Nightingale envisaged the well-being of mankind rather than the individual. Another reason may be that Welch's interest in Nightingale results from her 'involvement in the study and organization of the baccalaureate curriculum at St. Joseph's College, which is based upon Florence Nightingale's concepts' (Welch, p. 3). Given that, at present, curricula which are based on modern models of nursing emphasise the concept of the person so much, Welch could not but start to look for a concept of the active person in Nightingale's concept of nursing. Therefore, her point of departure was conducive to an interpretation of this concept of nursing being determined by the interpreter's needs rather than Nightingale's original works.

Environment
A further argument against the alleged emphasis on the person in Nightingale's concept of nursing lies in the major role attributed to the

environment, resulting in a concept of nursing that implied some sort of 'environmental engineering' rather than the idea of 'nursing the person'.

This conclusion is vindicated by the typically Nightingale combination of theology and science which was at the source of her position with regard to the controversy between miasmatism and contagionism. As pointed out earlier, the miasmatic position can be summarised as follows:

- whereas the environment is the active agent, the individual is attributed a passive role,
- medical treatment of epidemic disease is directed at manipulating the environmental causes rather than treating the individual affected by the disease,
- a universalistic attitude, implying that all relevant factors are interrelated and interdependent,
- the multicausal and interdependent explanation of disease.

As a result of Nightingale's taking sides with the miasmatists, her concept of nursing meets the criteria of what Ten Have (1983) called the sociological approach, as opposed to the biological approach, for miasmatism emphasises (Ten Have, 1983, p. 236):

the orientation towards the environmental variables, or the environment in the widest meaning of the word: society, the pattern of living, the circumstances of living, the culture as well as the water, the air and the soil.

As for Nightingale's concept of nursing, this sociological or environmentalist orientation should be taken to mean that:

- man's condition was subject to the circumstances affecting it,
- to change man's condition required the manipulation of the relevant circumstances, thereby changing the uniform relations between the individual and his environment,
- the uniform relations between man and his environment enabled man to govern his existence in accordance with the laws of nature which exemplified God's government of the world (universalistic attitude),
- man's condition was subject not only to the physical but also to the moral laws of nature (multicausal and interdependent explanation).

Another way of interpreting the environment in Nightingale's concept of nursing is the relevance of her views to the work of modern nursing theorists. Sister Callista Roy, for example, interprets it in terms of her own model of nursing (Roy, 1970, p. 44):

> *Florence Nightingale emphasized that contextual stimuli deal with environment.*

Apart from the fact that Nightingale never used the notion of contextual stimuli, Roy clearly overlooks the fact that the Nightingale's concept of nursing has nothing to do with her own notions of stress and adaptation whatsoever. Apart from that, it would appear that the notion of adaptation fits in better with the biological approach in so far as it emphasises the adaptational resources of the individual in relation to given environmental stimuli, and not vice versa.

Health

The third element to be evaluated concerns Nightingale's views on the nature of health and disease, the two modes of being she held to be equally subject to the laws of nature. However, because of the actual bifurcation of the field of nursing into hospital nursing, on the one hand, and district nursing, on the other, she nevertheless distinguished two branches of nursing, viz. nursing proper, or sick nursing, and health nursing, and by implication two sorts of nurses, viz. the sick nurse and the health-missioner. More importantly, though, both types of nurses had common ground in applying the self-same principles of sanitary science which constituted the laws of God with regard to the health of man's physical mode of being.

This interpretation is evidently at variance with that of others who refer to Nightingale's distinguishing sick nursing from health nursing as the basis for the distinction between hospital nursing and public health nursing (e.g. Seymer, 1954). The latter distinction, however, resulted not so much from Nightingale's concept of nursing as from the course of events in nursing practice. Indeed, long before the turn of the century, when institutional nursing became ancillary to both medicine and the hospital, nurse practitioners were drawn into the biological approach which became the increasingly dominant force in medicine, thereby giving rise to the image of the nurse who works under medical direction and provides physical care for the sick in the hospital. The health-missioner, on the other hand, was to become the 'visiting nurse', the forerunner of the public health nurse or health visitor, and this branch of nursing has always maintained close links with social work. So much so, that public health nursing, at times, came to be identified with 'social service' as opposed to 'institutional service' (Dock, 1912a, pp. 213–214).

As a result, and in contrast to the nurse practitioners in hospitals, public health nurses were also more aware of the importance of social factors in nursing practice.

However, the bifurcation of institutional and social service, as it emerged in the United States, was not implied by Nightingale's concept of nursing. To arrive at this bifurcation on the basis of Nightingale's writings on nursing is only possible by taking them at face value, and by refraining from an in-depth analysis of her concept of nursing which indicates that, in the final analysis, both sick nursing and health nursing amounted to a religiously-inspired, sanitary approach to nursing.

Nursing
Nightingale admittedly acknowledged that she used the word 'nursing' for want of a better one, and rightly so, for nursing in the sense of mothering or nurturing a child, or, for that matter, hospital nursing as it was known at the time, was not quite what she had in mind when using this word. For her, nursing was the art and science of applying sanitary principles, discovered by means of statistics, and manifesting God's law. Because of this ambiguity, the nursing actions which were outlined in her writings on nursing are open to two rather different interpretations.

One interpretation is based on the sanitary implications, the other on the religious presuppositions of her concept of nursing, and, with the notable exception of Welch (1986), most historians tend to go for the former rather than the latter interpretation. This is not to say that historians have failed to acknowledge Nightingale's interest in religious matters. However, only Welch goes so far as to contend that (Welch, 1986, p. 6):

> If *Suggestions for Thought* contains the foundations of her philosophy, then *Notes on Nursing* reflects the application of her philosophy.

To grasp the full meaning of Nightingale's concept of nursing, the interpretation must be based upon both its presuppositions and implications. For, in Nightingale's opinion, it was by helping the patient to live physically that the nurse helped him to develop and exercise his moral mode of being according to God's will as well. These moral aspects were essential to her concept of nursing.

Nursing education
The analysis of Nightingale's writings on nursing has shown her concept of nursing education to be a corollary of her concept of nursing. With regard to nursing education, Nightingale held the opinion that observation and reflection were to lead to the training and experience needed to

learn more and more about the character of God. On the other hand, Nightingale is known to have also been involved with the more down-to-earth matters involved in running a training school of nursing. Consequently, it is possible to interpret her writings on nursing education in two ways, either as a corollary of her concept of nursing or as reflecting her administrative involvement in running a training school. But it is the religious interpretation which most truly reflects Nightingale's thinking.

For example, when she stressed the need for special homes for nurses to enhance each nurse's 'esprit de corps' (Nightingale, 1882a and 1893), it was not so much an administrative measure to safeguard a place of living for nurses, as a way of enhancing the religious inspiration needed for the daily practice of nursing she hinted at.

Furthermore, Nightingale's writings on nursing education have given rise to interpretations which tell us more about the interpreter's frame of reference than Nightingale's. Barritt (1973, p. 10), for example, following the outcome of Newton's thesis (1949), uses Nightingale's religious beliefs to infer a human right to health and education:

> *These deep religious convictions made service to God her basic goal in life, according to Newton. To Miss Nightingale, serving God meant serving mankind. Since she believed that every human being had the right to health and to education, she made better health and better education her two objectives. The Nightingale Training School for Nurses embodied these two underlying aims that guided Miss Nightingale throughout her life.*

This interpretation, however, is suggestive of the struggle for professional education of nurses in the United States during the 20th century, rather than the religious pragmatism underlying Nightingale's concept of education.

Professional nursing

Finally, Nightingale's religious pragmatism was also the source of her opposition to the notion of a profession of nursing for, in her view, the nurse was called upon by God to acquire skills of observation and reflection in order to gain experience in applying the laws of health: this implied a life-long process of learning by experience and careful inquiry.

Notwithstanding the ample historical evidence corroborating this position of hers, not even Cook (1913a, p. 445) managed to escape from the conclusion that Nightingale not only 'recognized that nursing was an art and a science', but also that 'she raised it to the status of a profession'.

Worse still, Roberts (1937), although aware of Nightingale's position on this controversy, could not resist presenting her as being in favour of professionalisation by simply resorting to a definition of a profession that was not incompatible with Nightingale's notion of a calling – 'a vocation, by implication gainful, involving the individual and thoughtful application of a considerable body of organized knowledge in self-identifying service to others for the good of society' (1937, p. 775).

On the other hand, one of Nightingale's real contributions to nursing undoubtedly was (Smith, 1982, p. 155):

> to identify it in the public mind with sanctified duty. Contrary to nursing folklore, she neither invented modern nursing behaviour nor even the idea of nursing as a calling. But by bestowing her _imprimatur_ upon secular vocational nursing she gave it standing in Victorian Britain and throughout the world.

This contribution, however, appears to have had an inhibiting rather than a stimulating effect on the development of professional nursing, as nursing's image of 'sanctified duty' effectively pre-empted any efforts on the part of doctors, hospital administrators, and the general public, to meet the profession's demands for improvements in both nursing education and nursing practice.

One advantage of this ambivalent attitude towards nursing was that it has forced nurses to continuously identify and articulate their concept of professional nursing in order to achieve the profession's objectives.

Conclusion
As far as the conceptual development of nursing is concerned, there are two major reasons why Nightingale should not be seen as the founder of _modern_ nursing. One of the reasons has to do with the religious presuppositions of the Nightingale model of nursing, i.e. her religious pragmatism which has been shown to result in nothing less than a theological model of nursing; the other has to do with this model's sanitary implications. Between them, these presuppositions and implications resulted in a so-called sociological approach to nursing, as opposed to the biological approach (Ten Have, 1983).

As for the further development of modern nursing, the typically Nightingale combination of religious presuppositions and sanitary implications, as well as the sociological approach that went with it, have evidently failed to gain much support in modern nursing. In fact, history shows that nurses have gone their own way to the effect that the models of nursing to emerge, mainly in the United States, can not possibly have originated in the Nightingale model of nursing.

It is true to say that Nightingale's allegiance to miasmatism is now outdated and obsolete. Yet her sanitary principles live on to some extent in nursing today, albeit without its religious connotations. It is true to say that Nightingale's religious zeal and her imposition of this on nursing through a positive theology is inappropriate in today's secular profession of nursing. Yet the notion of a profession based on humanistic principles and a committment to caring (Watson, 1985) reflects a particular (if not unique) professional orientation, with elements of profession and calling within it, albeit not of a religious colouring. It is also true to say that the theory of modern nursing has outlived the ignorance reflected in miasmatism and sanitary laws.

Yet Nightingale's injunction to use knowledge in practice, and to reflect on practice from this knowledge base, is alive in the current theory-practice debate and the educational principles of reflective practice being actively pursued in modern nursing curricula. It can not be said, however, that there is an unbroken thread joining the elements of modern nursing to elements in Nightingale's thinking more than a century ago. Indeed, many of her ideas were long-forgotten or unknown to modern nurses and their relevance to modern nursing is, it may be argued, largely coincidental.

These conclusions raise the question of whether Nightingale's life and work have had any real significance in the development of modern nursing at all. This, it seems, is beyond doubt, albeit in the role of the living legend of nursing, which was reinforced by the image of the lady with the lamp rather than the founder of modern nursing. And, as for her image of the lady with the lamp, a legend cherished by so many of her biographers, it remains to be seen whether this image has not been detrimental rather than beneficial to the development of nursing. As one commentator (Baly, 1969, p. 4) states:

> ... *living in the shadow of a legend is not an unmitigated blessing. Exhorted to the 'Nightingale spirit', praised as 'ministering angels,' sicklied o'er with pale cast of sentimentality, nurses have tended to cling blindly to the tradition that raised them to such a pinnacle. To question the system was lèse-majesté, and this bred orthodoxy; conformity operates against reform. In spite of some enlightened questioning, the profession has tended to look back to its days of glory and has chosen not reform, but a crown of thorns.*

In the final analysis, nursing is still in the process of freeing itself from the bonds of servitude conjured up by the Nightingale myth. Also, as nursing builds a sound base of theory and practice, it has largely outlived the obsolete bases of Nightingale's model of nursing. However, in moving into the next century as a profession in its truest sense, with a sound body of knowledge and practice, nursing may yet be able to acknowledge and draw upon these aspects of the Nightingale legacy which still have relevance to modern nursing.

Bibliography

Agnew LRC (1958) Florence Nightingale – statistician. *American Journal of Nursing*, 58, 664–666.

Baly ME (1969) Florence Nightingale's influence on nursing today. *Nursing Times*, 65, (Jan. 2), Occ. Papers, pp. 1–4.

Baly ME (1984) *The influence of the Nightingale Fund from 1855 to 1914 on the development of nursing.* London, University of London, (unpublished doctoral thesis).

Baly ME (1986) *Florence Nightingale and the nursing legacy.* Beckenham (Kent), Croom Helm.

Baly ME (1986) Shattering the Nightingale myth. *Nursing Times*, 82, 16–19 (11 June).

Baly ME (1991) *As Miss Nightingale said...* London, Scutari Press.

Barritt ER (1973) Florence Nightingale's values and modern nursing education. *Nursing Forum*, 12, 7–48 (No. 1).

Bishop WJ (1957) Florence Nightingale's letters. *American Journal of Nursing*, 57, 607–610.

Bishop WJ (1960) Florence Nightingale's message for today. *Nursing Outlook*, 8, 246–250.

Bishop WJ & Goldie S (1962) *A bio-bibliography of Florence Nightingale.* London, Dawsons of Pall Mall, for the International Council of Nurses which is associated with the Florence Nightingale International Foundation.

Chinn PL & Kramer MK (1991) *Theory and nursing: a systematic approach.* St Louis, Mosby Year Book.

Cook E (1913a and 1913b) *The life of Florence Nightingale.* London, Macmillan and Co. (2 vols.).

Dewey J (1938) *Experience and education.* London, Collier-Macmillan Publishers.

Diamond M & Stone M (1981) Nightingale on Quetelet; I. The passionate statistician. *The Journal of the Royal Statistical Society*, 144, 66–79.

Dock LL (1912a and 1912b) *A history of nursing*. London, GP Putnam's Sons (Vols. III and IV).

Fawcett J (1984) The metaparadigm of nursing: present status and future refinements. *IMAGE: Journal of Nursing Scholarship*, 16, 84–87.

Fawcett J (1989) *Analysis and evaluation of conceptual models of nursing (2nd Edition)*. Philadelphia, FA Davis Company.

Fawcett J (1993) *Analysis and evaluation of nursing theories*. Philadelphia, FA Davis Company.

Goldie S (1980) *A calendar of the letters of Florence Nightingale*. Oxford, Oxford Microform Publications Ltd.

Goldie SM (1987) *Florence Nightingale in the Crimean War 1854–56*. Manchester, Manchester University Press.

Gordon R (1978) *The private life of Florence Nightingale*. New York, Atheneum Publishers.

Grier B & Grier M. (1978) Contributions of the passionate statistician. *Research in Nursing and Health*, 1, 103–109 (No. 3).

Hampton IA & others (1893) Educational standards for nurses. In: Hampton IA & others (1893) *Nursing of the sick*. Papers and discussions from the International Congress of Charities, Correction, and Philanthropy, Chicago, 1893. Reprinted under the sponsorship of the National League of Nursing Education. New York, McGraw-Hill Book Co., 1949, pp. 1–12.

Have H Ten (1983) *Geneeskunde en filosofie. De invloed van Jeremy Bentham op het medisch denken en handelen*. Lochem, De Tijdstroom.

Hebert RG (1981) *Florence Nightingale: saint, reformer or rebel?* Malabar (Flor.), Robert E. Krieger Publishing Company.

Henderson V (1966) *The nature of nursing: a definition and its implications for practice, research and education*. New York, Macmillan.

Huxley E (1975) *Florence Nightingale*. London, Weidenfeld and Nicholson.

Iveson-Iveson J. (1983) A legend in the breaking. *Nursing Mirror*, 11 May, 26–28.

Kalisch BJ & Kalisch PA (1983a) Heroine out of focus: media images of Florence Nightingale. Part I: Popular biographies and stage productions. *Nursing & Health Care* 4, 181–188.

Kalisch BJ & Kalisch PA (1983b) Heroine out of focus: media images of Florence Nightingale. Part II: Film, radio, and television dramatizations. *Nursing & Health Care*, 4, 270 – 279.

Kaplan A (1964) *The conduct of inquiry*. San Francisco, Chandler Publishing Company.

Kopf EW (1916) Florence Nightingale as a statistician. *Quarterly Publication of the American Statistical Association*, 15 (116), 388–404 (My source: *Research in Nursing and Health*, 1, 93–102 (No. 3).

Kuhn TS (1970) *The structure of scientific revolutions.* Chicago, University of Chicago Press.

Levine ME (1963) Florence Nightingale, the legend that lives. *Nursing Forum*, 2, 27–35 (No. 4).

Mantrip JC (1932) Florence Nightingale and religion. *London Quarterly and Holborn Review*, 318–325 (July).

Meleis A (1991) *Theoretical nursing: development and progress (2nd Edition).* New York, JB Lippincott Company.

Mills EW & Dale J (1964) Florence Nightingale and state registration. *International Nursing Review*, 11, 31–36 (No. 1).

Monteiro L (1972) Research into things past: tracking down one of Miss Nightingale's correspondents. *Nursing Research*, 21, 526–530.

Nash R (1914) *Florence Nightingale to her nurses.* New York, Macmillan.

Newton ME (1949) *Florence Nightingale's philosophy of life and education.* Stanford, University of California.

Newton ME (1965) The case for historical research. *Nursing Research*, 14, 20–27.

Nightingale F (1858) *Female nursing in military hospitals.* London, Harrisons and Sons, pp. 129–134.

Nightingale F (1859a) *Notes on hospitals.* London, Longman, Green, Longman, Roberts and Green, pp. 1–8.

Nightingale F (1859b) *Notes on nursing: what it is and what it is not.* London, G. Duckworth & Company Ltd 1970. (reprint).

Nightingale F (1860a) *Suggestions for thought to the searchers after truth among the artizans of England.* Vol. I. London, printed by George E. Eyre and William Spottiswoode.

Nightingale F (1860b) *Suggestions for thought to the searchers after religious truth.* Vol. II. London, printed by George E. Eyre and William Spottiswoode.

Nightingale F (1860c) *Suggestions for thought to the searchers after religious truth.* Vol. III. London, printed by George E. Eyre and William Spottiswoode.

Nightingale F (1865) *Organization of nursing in a large town.* London, Longman, Green, Reader and Dyer.

Nightingale F (1872) Florence Nightingale's letter of advice to Bellevue (September 18, 1872). *American Journal of Nursing*, 11, 361 – 364.

Nightingale F (1873a) A 'note' of interrogation. *Fraser's Magazine*, 7, 567–578.

Nightingale F (1873b) A 'subnote' of interrogation. I. What will be our religion in 1999? *Fraser's Magazine*, 8, 25–37.

Nightingale F (1882a) Nurses, training of. In: Seymer LR (1954) *Selected Writings of Florence Nightingale*. New York, Macmillan, pp. 319–334.

Nightingale F (1882b) Nursing the sick. In: Seymer LR (1954) *Selected Writings of Florence Nightingale*. New York, Macmillan, pp. 334–352.

Nightingale F (1892) *Health at home*. Winslow (Bucks), EJ French.

Nightingale F (1893) Sick nursing and health nursing. In: Hampton IA & others (1893) *Nursing of the sick*. New York, McGraw-Hill Book Co., 1949, pp. 24–43.

Nutting MA (1927) Florence Nightingale as statistician. *Public Health Nurse*, 19, 207–209.

Palmer IS (1977) Florence Nightingale: reformer, reactionary, researcher. *Nursing Research*, 26, 84–90.

Palmer IS (1983a) Florence Nightingale: the myth and the reality. *Nursing Times*, 79, 40–43 (Occ. Paper, No. 20).

Palmer IS (1983b) Nightingale revisited. *Nursing Outlook*, 31, 229–234.

Pickering G. (1974) *Creative malady*. London, George Allen & Unwin, pp. 99–178.

Poovey M (1991) *Cassandra and other selections from Suggestions for Thought*. London, Pickering and Chatto.

Prince J (1982) *Florence Nightingale's reform of nursing 1860-1887*. London, London School of Economics, (unpublished doctoral thesis).

Prince J (1984) Education for a profession: some lessons from history. *International Journal of Nursing Studies*, 21, 153–163.

Quain R (1895) *Dictionary of Medicine (2nd Edition)*. London.

Riehl JP & Roy C (1974) *Conceptual models for nursing practice*. New York, Appleton-Century-Crofts.

Roberts MM (1937) Florence Nightingale as a nurse educator. *American Journal of Nursing*, 37, 773–779.

Roy, Sister C (1970) Adaptation: a conceptual framework for nursing. *Nursing Outlook*. March, 18, 3, 42–45.

Schön DA (1983) *The Reflective Practitioner*. Temple Smith.

Schön DA (1987) *Educating the Reflective Practitioner*. San Francisco, Jossey-Bass.

Skretkowicz V (ed) (1992) *Florence Nightingale's Notes on Nursing (Revised with additions)*. London, Scutari Press.

Skretkowicz V (1993) Florence Nightingale's Notes on Nursing. *The Library*, 15, 1, 24–47.

Seymer LR (1954) *Selected Writings of Florence Nightingale.* New York, Macmillan.

Smith FB (1982) *Florence Nightingale. Reputation and power.* Beckenham (Kent), Croom Helm.

Smith FT (1981) Florence Nightingale: early feminist. *American Journal of Nursing*, 81, 1021–1025.

Stewart IM (1931) Trends in nursing education. *American Journal of Nursing*, 31, 601–612.

Stewart IM (1944) *The education of nurses. Historical foundations and modern trends.* New York, The Macmillan Company.

Strachey L (1918) *Eminent Victorians.* Chatto and Windus, London, pp. 115–177 (on Florence Nightingale). (My source is the issue of the Phoenix Library, dating from 1928).

Tarrant WG (1914) *Florence Nightingale as a religious thinker.* London, British and Foreign Unitarian Association. (The Unitarian Penny Library, No. 137).

Thompson JD (1980) The passionate humanist: from Nightingale to the new nurse. *Nursing Outlook*, 28, 290–296.

Vicinus M & Nergaard B (1989) *Ever Yours, Florence Nightingale.* London, Virago Press.

Watson J (1985) *Nursing: human science and health care.* Norwalk, Appleton-Century-Croft.

Welch M (1986) Nineteenth-century philosophic influences on Nightingale's concept of person. *Journal of Nursing History*, 1, 3–12 (No. 2).

Woodham-Smith C (1977) *Florence Nightingale 1820-1910.* London, Fontana Books.

Appendix:
Notes on Nursing

The text reproduced here has been photographically reproduced from the edition published in 1876 in London by Harrison. The quality of the type reflects the age of the original.

SHALL we begin by taking it as a general principle—that all disease, at some period or other of its course, is more or less a reparative process, not necessarily accompanied with suffering: an effort of nature to remedy a process of poisoning or of decay, which has taken place weeks, months, sometimes years beforehand, unnoticed, the termination of the disease being then, while the antecedent process was going on, determined? Disease a reparative process.

If we accept this as a general principle we shall be immediately met with anecdotes and instances to prove the contrary. Just so if we were to take, as a principle—all the climates of the earth are meant to be made habitable for man, by the efforts of man—the objection would be immediately raised,—Will the top of Mont Blanc ever be made habitable? Our answer would be, it will be many thousands of years before we have reached the bottom of Mont Blanc in making the earth healthy. Wait till we have reached the bottom before we discuss the top.

In watching disease, both in private houses and in public hospitals, the thing which strikes the experienced observer most forcibly is this, that the symptoms or the sufferings generally considered to be inevitable and incident to the disease are very often not symptoms of the disease at all, but of something quite different—of the want of fresh air, or of light, or of warmth, or of quiet, or of cleanliness, or of punctuality and care in the administration of diet, of each or of all of these. And this quite as much in private as in hospital nursing. Of the sufferings of disease, disease not always the cause.

The reparative process which Nature has instituted and which we call disease has been hindered by some want of knowledge or attention, in one or in all of these things, and pain, suffering, or interruption of the whole process sets in.

If a patient is cold, if a patient is feverish, if a patient is faint, if he is sick after taking food, if he has a bed-sore, it is generally the fault not of the disease, but of the nursing.

What nursing ought to do.

I use the word nursing for want of a better. It has been limited to signify little more than the administration of medicines and the application of poultices. It ought to signify the proper use of fresh air, light, warmth, cleanliness, quiet, and the proper selection and administration of diet—all at the least expense of vital power to the patient.

Nursing the sick little understood.

It has been said and written scores of times, that every woman makes a good nurse. I believe, on the contrary, that the very elements of nursing are all but unknown.

By this I do not mean that the nurse is always to blame. Bad sanitary, bad architectural, and bad administrative arrangements often make it impossible to nurse. But the art of nursing ought to include such arrangements as alone make what I understand by nursing, possible.

The art of nursing, as now practised, seems to be expressly constituted to unmake what God had made disease to be, viz., a reparative process.

Nursing ought to assist the reparative process.

To recur to the first objection. If we are asked, Is such or such a disease a reparative process? Can such an illness be unaccompanied with suffering? Will any care prevent such a patient from suffering this or that?—I humbly say, I do not know. But when you have done away with all that pain and suffering, which in patients are the symptoms not of their disease, but of the absence of one or all of the above-mentioned essentials to the success of Nature's reparative processes, we shall then know what are the symptoms of and the sufferings inseparable from the disease.

Another and the commonest exclamation which will be instantly made is—Would you do nothing, then, in cholera, fever, &c.?—so deep-rooted and universal is the conviction that to give medicine is to be doing something, or rather everything; to give air, warmth, cleanliness, &c., is to do nothing. The reply is, that in these and many other similar diseases the exact value of particular remedies and modes of treatment is by no means ascertained, while there is universal experience as to the extreme importance of careful nursing in determining the issue of the disease.

Nursing the well.

II. The very elements of what constitutes good nursing are as little understood for the well as for the sick. The same laws of health or of nursing, for they are in reality the same, obtain among the well as among the sick. The breaking of them produces only a less violent consequence among the former than among the latter,—and this sometimes, not always.

It is constantly objected,—"But how can I obtain this medical knowledge? I am not a doctor. I must leave this to doctors."

Little understood.

Oh, mothers of families! You who say this, do you know that one in every seven infants in this civilized land of England perishes before it is one year old? That, in London, two in every five die before they are five years old? And, in the other great cities of

England, nearly one out of two?* "The life duration of tender babies" (as some Saturn, turned analytical chemist, says) "is the most delicate test" of sanitary conditions. Is all this premature suffering and death necessary? Or did Nature intend mothers to be always accompanied by doctors? Or is it better to learn the piano-forte than to learn the laws which subserve the preservation of offspring?

Macaulay somewhere says, that it is extraordinary that, whereas the laws of the motions of the heavenly bodies, far removed as they are from us, are perfectly well understood, the laws of the human mind, which are under our observation all day and every day, are no better understood than they were two thousand years ago.

But how much more extraordinary is it that, whereas what we might call the coxcombries of education—e.g., the elements of astronomy—are now taught to every school-girl, neither mothers of families of any class, nor school-mistresses of any class, nor nurses of children, nor nurses of hospitals, are taught anything about those laws which God has assigned to the relations of our bodies with the world in which He has put them. In other words, the laws which make these bodies, into which He has put our minds, healthy or unhealthy organs of those minds, are all but unlearnt. Not but that these laws—the laws of life—are in a certain measure understood, but not even mothers think it worth their while to study them—to study how to give their children healthy existences. They call it medical or physiological knowledge, fit only for doctors.

Another objection.

We are constantly told,—"But the circumstances which govern our children's healths are beyond our control. What can we do with winds? There is the east wind. Most people can tell before they get up in the morning whether the wind is in the east."

* Upon this fact the most wonderful deductions have been strung. For a long time an announcement something like the following has been going the round of the papers:—"More than 25,000 children die every year in London under 10 years of age; therefore we want a Children's Hospital." This spring there was a prospectus issued, and divers other means taken to this effect:— "There is a great want of sanitary knowledge in women; therefore we want a Women's Hospital." Now, both the above facts are too sadly true. But what is the deduction? The causes of this enormous child mortality are perfectly well known; they are chiefly want of cleanliness, want of ventilation, want of whitewashing; in one word, defective *household* hygiene. The remedies are just as well known; and among them is certainly not the establishment of a Child's Hospital. This may be a want; just as there may be a want of hospital room for adults. But the Registrar-General would certainly never think of giving us as a cause for the high rate of child mortality in (say) Liverpool that there was not sufficient hospital room for children; nor would he urge upon us, as a remedy, to found a hospital for them.

Again, women, and the best women, are wofully deficient in sanitary knowledge; although it is to women that we must look, first and last, for its application, as far as *household* hygiene is concerned. But who would ever think of citing the institution of a Women's Hospital as the way to cure this want?

We have it, indeed, upon very high authority that there is some fear lest hospitals, as they have been *hitherto*, may not have generally increased, rather than diminished, the rate of mortality—especially of child mortality.

Curious deductions from an excessive death rate.

To this one can answer with more certainty than to the former objections. Who is it who knows when the wind is in the east? Not the Highland drover, certainly, exposed to the east wind, but the young lady who is worn out with the want of exposure to fresh air, to sunlight, &c. Put the latter under as good sanitary circumstances as the former, and she too will not know when the wind is in the east.

I. VENTILATION AND WARMING.

First rule of nursing, to keep the air within as pure as the air without.

The very first canon of nursing, the first and the last thing upon which a nurse's attention must be fixed, the first essential to the patient, without which all the rest you can do for him is as nothing, with which I had almost said you may leave all the rest alone, is this: TO KEEP THE AIR HE BREATHES AS PURE AS THE EXTERNAL AIR, WITHOUT CHILLING HIM. Yet what is so little attended to? Even where it is thought of at all, the most extraordinary misconceptions reign about it. Even in admitting air into the patient's room or ward, few people ever think, where that air comes from. It may come from a corridor into which other wards are ventilated, from a hall, always unaired, always full of the fumes of gas, dinner, of various kinds of mustiness; from an underground kitchen, sink, washhouse, water-closet, or even, as I myself have had sorrowful experience, from open sewers loaded with filth; and with this the patient's room or ward is aired, as it is called—poisoned, it should rather be said. Always air from the air without, and that, too, through those windows, through which the air comes freshest. From a closed court, especially if the wind do not blow that way, air may come as stagnant as any from a hall or corridor.

Again, a thing I have often seen both in private houses and institutions. A room remains uninhabited; the fire place is carefully fastened up with a board; the windows are never opened; probably the shutters are kept always shut; perhaps some kind of stores are kept in the room; no breath of fresh air can by possibility enter into that room, nor any ray of sun. The air is as stagnant, musty, and corrupt as it can by possibility be made. It is quite ripe to breed small-pox, scarlet fever, diphtheria, or anything else you please.*

Yet the nursery, ward, or sick room adjoining will positively be aired (?) by having the door opened into that room. Or children will be put into that room, without previous preparation, to sleep.

A short time ago a man walked into a back-kitchen in Queen

Why are uninhabited rooms shut up?

* The common idea as to uninhabited rooms is, that they may safely be left with doors, windows, shutters, and chimney board, all closed—hermetically sealed if possible—to keep out the dust, it is said; and that no harm will happen if the room is but opened a short hour before the inmates are put in. I have often been asked the question for uninhabited rooms.—But when ought the windows to be opened? The answer is—When ought they to be shut?

square, and cut the throat of a poor consumptive creature, sitting by the fire. The murderer did not deny the act, but simply said, "It's all right." Of course he was mad.

But in our case, the extraordinary thing is that the victim says, "It's all right," and that we are not mad. Yet, although we "nose" the murderers, in the musty unaired unsunned room, the scarlet fever which is behind the door, or the fever and hospital gangrene which are stalking among the crowded beds of a hospital ward, we say, "It's all right."

With a proper supply of windows, and a proper supply of fuel in open fire places, fresh air is comparatively easy to secure when your patient or patients are in bed. Never be afraid of open windows then. People don't catch cold in bed. This is a popular fallacy. With proper bed-clothes and hot bottles, if necessary, you can always keep a patient warm in bed, and well ventilate him at the same time. *Without chill.*

But a careless nurse, be her rank and education what it may, will stop up every cranny and keep a hot-house heat when her patient is in bed,—and, if he is able to get up, leave him comparatively unprotected. The time when people take cold (and there are many ways of taking cold, besides a cold in the nose,) is when they first get up after the two-fold exhaustion of dressing and of having had the skin relaxed by many hours, perhaps days, in bed, and thereby rendered more incapable of re-action. Then the same temperature which refreshes the patient in bed may destroy the patient just risen. And common sense will point out that, while purity of air is essential, a temperature must be secured which shall not chill the patient. Otherwise the best that can be expected will be a feverish re-action.

To have the air within as pure as the air without, it is not necessary, as often appears to be thought, to make it as cold.

In the afternoon again, without care, the patient whose vital powers have then risen often finds the room as close and oppressive as he found it cold in the morning. Yet the nurse will be terrified, if a window is opened*.

I know an intelligent humane house surgeon who makes a practice of keeping the ward windows open. The physicians and surgeons invariably close them while going their rounds; and the house surgeon very properly as invariably opens them whenever the doctors have turned their backs. *Open windows.*

In a little book on nursing, published a short time ago, we are told, that "with proper care it is very seldom that the windows cannot be opened for a few minutes twice in the day to admit fresh

* It is very desirable that the windows in a sick room should be such as that the patient shall, if he can move about, be able to open and shut them easily himself. In fact the sick room is very seldom kept aired if this is not the case—so very few people have any perception of what is a healthy atmosphere for the sick. The sick man often says, "This room where I spend 22 hours out of the 24 is fresher than the other where I only spend 2. Because here I can manage the windows myself." And it is true.

air from without." I should think not; nor twice in the hour either. It only shows how little the subject has been considered.

What kind of warmth desirable. Of all methods of keeping patients warm the very worst certainly is to depend for heat on the breath and bodies of the sick. I have known a medical officer keep his ward windows hermetically closed, thus exposing the sick to all the dangers of an infected atmosphere, because he was afraid that, by admitting fresh air, the temperature of the ward would be too much lowered. This is a destructive fallacy.

To attempt to keep a ward warm at the expense of making the sick repeatedly breathe their own hot, humid, putrescing atmosphere is a certain way to delay recovery or to destroy life.

Bedrooms almost universally foul. Do you ever go into the bed-rooms of any persons of any class, whether they contain one, two, or twenty people, whether they hold sick or well, at night, or before the windows are opened in the morning, and ever find the air anything but unwholesomely close and foul? And why should it be so? And of how much importance it is that it should not be so? During sleep, the human body, even when in health, is far more injured by the influence of foul air than when awake. Why can't you keep the air all night, then, as pure as the air without in the rooms you sleep in? But for this, you must have sufficient outlet for the impure air you make yourselves to go out; sufficient inlet for the pure air from without to come in. You must have open chimneys, open windows, or ventilators; no close curtains round your beds; no shutters or curtains to your windows, none of the contrivances by which you undermine your own health or destroy the chances of recovery of your sick.*

An air-test of essential consequence. * Dr. Angus Smith's air test, if it could be made of simpler application, would be invaluable to use in every sleeping and sick room. Just as without the use of a thermometer no nurse should ever put a patient into a bath, so should no nurse, or mother, or superintendent be without the air test in any ward, nursery, or sleeping-room. If the main function of a nurse is to maintain the air within the room as fresh as the air without, without lowering the temperature, then she should always be provided with a thermometer which indicates the temperature, with an air-test which indicates the organic matter of the air. But to be used, the latter must be made as simple a little instrument as the former, and both should be self-registering. The senses of nurses and mothers become so dulled to foul air that they are perfectly unconscious of what an atmosphere they have let their children, patients, or charges, sleep in. But if the tell-tale air-test were to exhibit in the morning, both to nurses and patients and to the superior officer going round, what the atmosphere has been during the night, I question if any greater security could be afforded against a recurrence of the misdemeanour.

And oh; the crowded national school! where so many children's epidemics have their origin, what a tale its air-test would tell! We should have parents saying, and saying rightly, "I will not send my child to that school, the air-test stands at 'Horrid.'" And the dormitories of our great boarding schools! Scarlet fever would be no more ascribed to contagion, but to its right cause, the air-test standing at "Foul."

We should hear no longer of "Mysterious Dispensations," and of "Plague and Pestilence," being "in God's hands," when, so far as we know, He has put them into our own. The little air-test would both betray the cause of these "mysterious pestilences," and call upon us to remedy it.

A careful nurse will keep a constant watch over her sick, especially weak, protracted, and collapsed cases, to guard against the effects of the loss of vital heat by the patient himself. In certain diseased states much less heat is produced than in health; and there is a constant tendency to the decline and ultimate extinction of the vital powers by the call made upon them to sustain the heat of the body. Cases where this occurs should be watched with the greatest care from hour to hour, I had almost said from minute to minute. The feet and legs should be examined by the hand from time to time, and whenever a tendency to chilling is discovered, hot bottles, hot bricks, or warm flannels, with some warm drink, should be made use of until the temperature is restored. The fire should be, if necessary, replenished. Patients are frequently lost in the latter stages of disease from want of attention to such simple precautions. The nurse may be trusting to the patient's diet, or to his medicine, or to the occasional dose of stimulant which she is directed to give him, while the patient is all the while sinking from want of a little external warmth. Such cases happen at all times, even during the height of summer. This fatal chill is most apt to occur towards early morning at the period of the lowest temperature of the twenty-four hours, and at the time when the effect of the preceding day's diets is exhausted.

When warmth must be most carefully looked to.

Generally speaking, you may expect that weak patients will suffer cold much more in the morning than in the evening. The vital powers are much lower. If they are feverish at night, with burning hands and feet, they are almost sure to be chilly and shivering in the morning. But nurses are very fond of heating the foot-warmer at night, and of neglecting it in the morning, when they are busy. I should reverse the matter.

All these things require common sense and care. Yet perhaps in no one single thing is so little common sense shewn, in all ranks, as in nursing.*

The extraordinary confusion between cold and ventilation, in the minds of even well educated people, illustrates this. To make a room cold is by no means necessarily to ventilate it. Nor is it at all necessary, in order to ventilate a room, to chill it. Yet, if a nurse finds a room close, she will let out the fire, thereby making it closer, or she will open the door into a cold room, without a fire, or an open window in it, by way of improving the ventilation.

Cold air not ventilation, nor fresh air a method of chill.

* With private sick, I think, but certainly with hospital sick, the nurse should never be satisfied as to the freshness of their atmosphere, unless she can feel the air gently moving over her face, when still.

But it is often observed that nurses who make the greatest outcry against open windows are those who take the least pains to prevent dangerous draughts. The door of the patients' room or ward *must* sometimes stand open to allow of persons passing in and out, or heavy things being carried in and out. The careful nurse will keep the door shut while she shuts the windows, and then, and not before, set the door open, so that a patient may not be left sitting up in bed, perhaps in a profuse perspiration, directly in the draught between the open door and window. Neither, of course, should a patient, while being washed or in any way exposed, remain in the draught of an open window or door.

[Original page no. 11]

The safest atmosphere of all for a patient is a good fire and an open window, excepting in extremes of temperature. (Yet no nurse can ever be made to understand this.) To ventilate a small room without draughts of course requires more care than to ventilate a large one.

Night air.

Another extraordinary fallacy is the dread of night air. What air can we breathe at night but night air? The choice is between pure night air from without and foul night air from within. Most people prefer the latter. An unaccountable choice. What will they say if it is proved to be true that fully one-half of all the disease we suffer from is occasioned by people sleeping with their windows shut? An open window most nights in the year can never hurt any one. This is not to say that light is not necessary for recovery. In great cities, night air is often the best and purest air to be had in the twenty-four hours. I could better understand in towns shutting the windows during the day than during the night, for the sake of the sick. The absence of smoke, the quiet, all tend to making night the best time for airing the patients. One of our highest medical authorities on Consumption and Climate has told me that the air in London is never so good as after ten o'clock at night.

Air from the outside. Open your windows, shut your doors.

Always air your room, then, from the outside air, if possible. Windows are made to open; doors are made to shut—a truth which seems extremely difficult of apprehension. I have seen a careful nurse airing her patient's room through the door, near to which were two gaslights, (each of which consumes as much air as eleven men), a kitchen, a corridor, the composition of the atmosphere in which consisted of gas, paint, foul air, never changed, full of effluvia, including a current of sewer air from an ill-placed sink, ascending in a continual stream by a well-staircase, and discharging themselves constantly into the patient's room. The window of the said room, if opened, was all that was desirable to air it. Every room must be aired from without—every passage from without. But the fewer passages there are in a hospital the better.

Smoke.

If we are to preserve the air within as pure as the air without, it is needless to say that the chimney must not smoke. Almost all smoky chimneys can be cured—from the bottom, not from the top. Often it is only necessary to have an inlet for air to supply the fire, which is feeding itself, for want of this, from its own chimney. On the other hand, almost all chimneys can be made to smoke by a careless nurse, who lets the fire get low and then overwhelms it with coal; not, as we verily believe, in order to spare herself trouble, (for very rare is unkindness to the sick), but from not thinking what she is about.

Airing damp things in a patient's room.

In laying down the principle that the first object of the nurse must be to keep the air breathed by her patient as pure as the air without, it must not be forgotten that everything in the room which can give off effluvia, besides the patient, evaporates itself into his air. And it follows that there ought to be nothing in the room, excepting him, which can give off effluvia or moisture. Out of all damp towels, &c., which become dry in the room, the damp, of course, goes into the patient's air. Yet this "of course" seems as little thought of, as if it were an obsolete fiction. How very seldom you see a nurse who acknowledges by her practice that nothing at all ought to be aired in the patient's room, that nothing at all ought to be cooked at the patient's fire! Indeed the arrangements often make this rule impossible to observe.

If the nurse be a very careful one, she will, when the patient leaves his bed, but not his room, open the sheets wide, and throw the bed clothes back, in order to air his bed. And she will spread the wet towels or flannels carefully out upon a horse, in order to dry them. Now either these bed-clothes and towels are not dried and aired, or they dry and air themselves into the patient's air. And whether the damp and effluvia do him most harm in his air or in his bed, I leave to you to determine, for I cannot.

Even in health people cannot repeatedly breathe air in which **Effluvia from** they live with impunity, on account of its becoming charged with **excreta.** unwholesome matter from the lungs and skin. In disease where everything given off from the body is highly noxious and dangerous, not only must there be plenty of ventilation to carry off the effluvia, but everything which the patient passes must be instantly removed away, as being more noxious than even the emanations from the sick.

Of the fatal effects of the effluvia from the excreta it would seem unnecessary to speak, were they not so constantly neglected. Concealing the utensils behind the vallance to the bed seems all the precaution which is thought necessary for safety in private nursing. Did you but think for one moment of the atmosphere under that bed, the saturation of the under side of the mattress with the warm evaporations, you would be startled and frightened too!

The use of any chamber utensil *without a lid** should be utterly **Chamber uten-** abolished, whether among sick or well. You can easily convince **sils without** yourself of the necessity of this absolute rule, by taking one with a **lids.**

---

* But never, never should the possession of this indispensable lid confirm you **Don't make** in the abominable practice of letting the chamber utensil remain in a patient's **your sick-room** room unemptied, except once in the 24 hours, *i.e.*, when the bed is made. Yes, **into a sewer.** impossible as it may appear, I have known the best and most attentive nurses guilty of this; aye, and have known, too, a patient afflicted with severe diarrhœa for ten days, and the nurse (a very good one) not know of it, because the chamber utensil (one with a lid) was emptied only once in the 24 hours, and that by the housemaid who came in and made the patient's bed every evening. As well might you have a sewer under the room, or think that in a water closet the plug need be pulled up but once a day. Also take care that your *lid*, as well as your utensil, be always thoroughly rinsed.

If a nurse declines to do these kinds of things for her patient, "because it is not her business," I should say that nursing was not her calling. I have seen surgical "sisters," women whose hands were worth to them two or three guineas a-week, down upon their knees scouring a room or hut, because they thought it otherwise not fit for their patients to go into. I am far from wishing nurses to scour. It is a waste of power. But I do say that these women had the true nurse-calling—the good of their sick first, and second only the consideration what it was their "place" to do—and that women who wait for the housemaid to do this, or for the charwoman to do that, when their patients are suffering, have not the *making* of a nurse in them.

[Original page no. 13]

lid, and examining the under side of that lid. It will be found always covered, whenever the utensil is not empty, by condensed offensive moisture. Where does that go, when there is no lid?

Earthenware, or if there is any wood, highly polished and varnished wood, are the only materials fit for patients' utensils. The very lid of the old abominable close-stool is enough to breed a pestilence. It becomes saturated with offensive matter, which scouring is only wanted to bring out. I prefer an earthenware lid as being always cleaner. But there are various good new-fashioned arrangements.

Abolish slop-pails.

A slop-pail should never be brought into a sick room. It should be a rule invariable, rather more important in the private house than elsewhere, that the utensil should be carried directly to the water-closet, emptied there, rinsed there, and brought back. There should always be water and a cock in every water-closet for rinsing. But even if there is not, you must carry water there to rinse with. I have actually seen, in the private sick room, the utensils emptied into the foot-pan, and put back unrinsed under the bed. I can hardly say which is most abominable, whether to do this or to rinse the utensil *in* the sick room. In the best hospitals it is now a rule that no slop-pail shall ever be brought into the wards, but that the utensils shall be carried direct to be emptied and rinsed at the proper place. I would it were so in the private house.

Fumigations.

Let no one ever depend upon fumigations, "disinfectants," and the like, for purifying the air. The offensive thing, not its smell, must be removed. A celebrated medical lecturer began one day "Fumigations, gentlemen, are of essential importance. They make such an abominable smell that they compel you to open the window." I wish all the disinfecting fluids invented made such an "abominable smell" that they forced you to admit fresh air. That would be a useful invention.

II.—HEALTH OF HOUSES*.

Health of houses. Five points essential.

There are five essential points in securing the health of houses:—

1. Pure air.
2. Pure water.
3. Efficient drainage.
4. Cleanliness.
5. Light.

Health of carriages.

* The health of carriages, especially close carriages, is not of sufficient universal importance to mention here, otherwise than cursorily. Children, who are always the most delicate test of sanitary conditions, generally cannot enter a close carriage without being sick—and very lucky for them that it is so. A close carriage, with the horse-hair cushions and linings always saturated with organic matter, if to this be added the windows up, is one of the most unhealthy of human receptacles. The idea of taking an *airing* in it is something preposterous. Dr. Angus Smith has shown that a crowded railway carriage, which goes at the rate of 30 miles an hour, is as unwholesome as the strong smell of a sewer, or as a back yard in one of the most unhealthy courts off one of the most unhealthy streets in Manchester.

Without these, no house can be healthy. And it will be unhealthy just in proportion as they are deficient.

1. To have pure air, your house must be so constructed as that the Pure air. outer atmosphere shall find its way with ease to every corner of it. House architects hardly ever consider this. The object in building a house is to obtain the largest interest for the money, not to save doctors' bills to the tenants. But, if tenants should ever become so wise as to refuse to occupy unhealthily constructed houses, and if Insurance Companies should ever come to understand their interest so thoroughly as to pay a Sanitary Surveyor to look after the houses where their clients live, speculative architects would speedily be brought to their senses. As it is, they build what pays best. And there are always people foolish enough to take the houses they build. And if in the course of time the families die off, as is so often the case, nobody ever thinks of blaming any but Providence* for the result. Ill-informed medical men aid in sustaining the delusion, by laying the blame on "current contagions." Badly constructed houses do for the healthy what badly constructed hospitals do for the sick. Once insure that the air in a house is stagnant, and sickness is certain to follow.

2. Pure water is more generally introduced into houses than it Pure water. used to be, thanks to the exertions of the sanitary reformers. Within the last few years, a large part of London was in the daily habit of using water polluted by the drainage of its sewers and water closets. This has happily been remedied. But, in many parts of the country, well water of a very impure kind is used for domestic purposes. And when epidemic disease shows itself, persons using such water are almost sure to suffer.

3. It would be curious to ascertain by inspection, how many Drainage. houses in London are really well drained. Many people would say, surely all or most of them. But many people have no idea in what good drainage consists. They think that a sewer in the street, and a pipe leading to it from the house is good drainage. All the while the sewer may be nothing but a laboratory from which epidemic disease and ill health is being distilled into the house. No house with any untrapped drain pipe communicating immediately with a sewer, whether it be from water closet, sink, or gully-grate, can ever be healthy. An untrapped sink may at any time spread fever or pyæmia among the inmates of a palace.

The ordinary oblong sink is an abomination. That great surface Sinks. of stone, which is always left wet, is always exhaling into the air. I have known whole houses and hospitals smell of the sink. I have met just as strong a stream of sewer air coming up the back staircase of a grand London house from the sink, as I have ever met at

* God lays down certain physical laws. Upon His carrying out such laws depends our responsibility (that much abused word), for how could we have any responsibility for actions, the results of which we could not foresee—which would be the case if the carrying out of His laws were *not* certain. Yet we seem to be continually expecting that He will work a miracle—*i. e.* break His own laws expressly to relieve us of responsibility.

[Original page no. 15]

Scutari; and I have seen the rooms in that house all ventilated by the open doors, and the passages all *un*ventilated by the closed windows, in order that as much of the sewer air as possible might be conducted into and retained in the bed-rooms. It is wonderful.

Another great evil in house construction is carrying drains underneath the house. Such drains are never safe. All house drains should begin and end outside the walls. Many people will readily admit, as a theory, the importance of these things. But how few are there who can intelligently trace disease in their households to such causes! Is it not a fact, that when scarlet fever, measles, or small-pox appear among the children, the very first thought which occurs is, "where" the children can have "caught" the disease? And the parents immediately run over in their minds all the families with whom they may have been. They never think of looking at home for the source of the mischief. If a neighbour's child is seized with small pox, the first question which occurs is whether it had been vaccinated. No one would undervalue vaccination; but it becomes of doubtful benefit to society when it leads people to look abroad for the source of evils which exist at home.

Cleanliness.

4. Without cleanliness, within and without your house, ventilation is comparatively useless. In certain foul districts of London, poor people used to object to open their windows and doors because of the foul smells that came in. Rich people like to have their stables and dunghill near their houses. But does it ever occur to them that with many arrangements of this kind it would be safer to keep the windows shut than open? You cannot have the air of the house pure with dung heaps under the windows. These are common all over London. And yet people are surprised that their children, brought up in large "well-aired" nurseries and bed-rooms suffer from children's epidemics. If they studied Nature's laws in the matter of children's health, they would not be so surprised.

There are other ways of having filth inside a house besides having dirt in heaps. Old papered walls of years' standing, dirty carpets, uncleansed furniture, are just as ready sources of impurity to the air as if there were a dung-heap in the basement. People are so unaccustomed from education and habits to consider how to make a home healthy, that they either never think of it at all, and take every disease as a matter of course, to be "resigned to" when it comes "as from the hand of Providence;" or if they ever entertain the idea of preserving the health of their household as a duty, they are very apt to commit all kinds of "negligences and ignorances" in performing it.

Light.

5. A dark house is always an unhealthy house, always an ill-aired house, always a dirty house. Want of light stops growth, and promotes scrofula, rickets, &c., among the children.

People lose their health in a dark house, and if they get ill they cannot get well again in it. More will be said about this farther on.

Three common errors in managing the health of houses.

Three out of many "negligences and ignorances" in managing the health of houses generally, I will here mention as specimens—1. That the female head in charge of any building does not think it necessary to visit every hole and corner of it every day. How can she expect those who are under her to be more careful to maintain her house in a healthy condition than she who is in charge of it?—2. That it is not considered essential to air, to sun, and to clean rooms while uninhabited; which is simply ignoring the first elementary notion of sanitary things, and laying the ground ready for all kinds of diseases.—3. That the window, and one window, is considered enough to air a room. Have you never observed that any room without a fire-place is always close? And, if you have a fire-place, would you cram it up not only with a chimney-board, but perhaps with a great wisp of brown paper, in the throat of the chimney—to prevent the soot from coming down, you say? If your chimney is foul, sweep it; but don't expect that you can ever air a room with only one aperture; don't suppose that to shut up a room is the way to keep it clean. It is the best way to foul the room and all that is in it. Don't imagine that if you, who are in charge, don't look to all these things yourself, those under you will be more careful than you are. It appears as if the part of a mistress now is to complain of her servants, and to accept their excuses—not to show them how there need be neither complaints made nor excuses.

But again, to look to all these things yourself does not mean to do them yourself. "I always open the windows," the head in charge often says. If you do it, it is by so much the better, certainly, than if it were not done at all. But can you not insure that it is done when not done by yourself? Can you insure that it is not undone when your back is turned? This is what being "in charge" means. And a very important meaning it is, too. The former only implies that just what you can do with your own hands is done. The latter that what ought to be done is always done. *Head in charge must see to House Hygiene, not do it herself.*

And now, you think these things trifles, or at least exaggerated. But what you "think" or what I "think" matters little. Let us see what God thinks of them. God always justifies His ways. While we are thinking, He has been teaching. I have known cases of hospital pyæmia quite as severe in handsome private houses as in any of the worst hospitals, and from the same cause, viz., foul air. Yet nobody learnt the lesson. Nobody learnt *anything* at all from it. They went on *thinking*—thinking that the sufferer had scratched his thumb, or that it was singular that "all the servants" had "whitlows," or that something was "much about this year; there is always sickness in our house." This is a favourite mode of thought—leading *not* to inquire what is the uniform cause of these general "whitlows," but to stifle all inquiry. In what sense is "sickness" being "always there," a justification of its being "there" at all? *Does God think of these things so seriously?*

I will tell you what was the cause of this hospital pyæmia being in that large private house. It was that the sewer air from an ill-placed sink was carefully conducted into all the rooms by sedulously opening all the doors, and closing all the passage windows. It was that the slops were emptied into the foot pans;—it was that the utensils were never properly rinsed;—it was that the chamber *How does He carry out His laws?*

crockery was rinsed with dirty water;—it was that the beds were never properly shaken, aired, picked to pieces, or changed. It was that the carpets and curtains were always musty;—it was that the furniture was always dusty; it was that the papered walls were saturated with dirt;—it was that the floors were never cleaned;—it was that the uninhabited rooms were never sunned, or cleaned, or aired; —it was that the cupboards were always reservoirs of foul air;—it was that the windows were always tight shut up at night;—it was that no window was ever systematically opened, even in the day, or that the right window was not opened. A person gasping for air might open a window for himself. But the servants were not taught to open the windows, to shut the doors; or they opened the windows upon a dank well between high walls, not upon the airier court; or they opened the room doors into the unaired halls and passages, by way of airing the rooms. Now all this is not fancy, but fact.

How does He teach His laws? In that handsome house I have known in one summer three cases of hospital pyæmia, one of phlebitis, two of consumptive cough : all the *immediate* products of foul air. When, in temperate climates, a house is more unhealthy in summer than in winter, it is a certain sign of something wrong. Yet nobody learns the lesson. Yes, God always justifies His ways. He is teaching while you are not learning. This poor body loses his finger, that one loses his life. And all from the most easily preventible causes.*

Physical degeneration in families. Its causes. The houses of the grandmothers and great grandmothers of this generation, at least the country houses, with front door and back door always standing open, winter and summer, and a thorough draught always blowing through—with all the scrubbing, and cleaning, and polishing, and scouring which used to go on, the grandmothers, and still more the great grandmothers, always out of doors and never with a bonnet on except to go to church, these things entirely account for the fact so often seen of a great grandmother, who was a tower of physical vigour descending into a grandmother perhaps a little less vigorous but still sound as a bell and healthy to the core, into a mother languid and confined to her carriage and house, and lastly into a daughter sickly and confined to her bed. For, remember, even with a general decrease of mortality you may often find a race thus degenerating and still oftener a family. You may see poor little feeble washed-out rags, children of a noble stock, suffering morally and physically, throughout their useless, degenerate

Servants' rooms. * I must say a word about servants' bed-rooms. From the way they are built, but oftener from the way they are kept, and from no intelligent inspection whatever being exercised over them, they are almost invariably dens of foul air, and the "servants' health" suffers in an "unaccountable" (?) way, even in the country. For I am by no means speaking only of London houses, where too often servants are put to live under the ground and over the roof. But in a country *"mansion,"* which was really a "mansion," (not after the fashion of advertisements), I have known three maids who slept in the same room ill of scarlet fever. "How catching it is," was of course the remark. One look at the room, one smell of the room, was quite enough. It was no longer "unaccountable." The room was not a small one; it was up stairs, and it had two large windows—but nearly every one of the neglects enumerated above was there.

lives, and yet people who are going to marry and to bring more such into the world, will consult nothing but their own convenience as to where they are to live, or how they are to live.

With regard to the health of houses where there is a sick person, it often happens that the sick room is made a ventilating shaft for the rest of the house. For while the house is kept as close, unaired, and dirty as usual, the window of the sick room is kept a little open always, and the door occasionally. Now, there are certain sacrifices which a house with one sick person in it does make to that sick person: it ties up its knocker; it lays straw before it in the street. Why can't it keep itself thoroughly clean and unusually well aired, in deference to the sick person?

We must not forget what, in ordinary language, is called "Infection;" *—a thing of which people are generally so afraid that they frequently follow the very practice in regard to it which they ought to avoid. Nothing used to be considered so infectious or contagious as small pox; and people not very long ago used to cover up patients with heavy bed clothes, while they kept up large fires and shut the windows. Small pox, of course, under this *régime*, is very "infectious." People are somewhat wiser now in their management of this disease. They have ventured to cover the patients lightly and to keep the windows open; and we hear much less of the "infection" of small pox than we used to do. But do people in our days act with more wisdom on the subject of "infection" in fevers—scarlet fever, measles, &c.—than their forefathers did with small pox? Does not the popular idea of "infection" involve that people should take greater care of themselves than of the patient? that, for instance, it is safer not to be too much with the patient, not to attend too much to his wants? Perhaps the best illustration of the utter absurdity of this view of duty in attending on "infectious" diseases is afforded by what was very recently the practice, if it is

Don't make your sick-room into a ventilating shaft for the whole house.

Infection.

* Is it not living in a continual mistake to look upon diseases, as we do now, as separate entities, which *must* exist, like cats and dogs? instead of looking upon them as conditions, like a dirty and a clean condition, and just as much under our own control; or rather as the reactions of kindly nature, against the conditions in which we have placed ourselves.

Diseases are not individuals arranged in classes, like cats and dogs,

I was brought up, both by scientific men and ignorant women, distinctly to believe that small-pox, for instance, was a thing of which there was once a first specimen in the world, which went on propagating itself, in a perpetual chain of descent, just as much as that there was a first dog, (or a first pair of dogs), and that small-pox would not begin itself any more than a new dog would begin without there having been a parent dog.

but conditions growing out of one another.

Since then I have seen with my eyes and smelt with my nose small-pox growing up in first specimens, either in close rooms or in overcrowded wards, where it could not by any possibility have been "caught," but must have begun.

Nay, more, I have seen diseases begin, grow up, and pass into one another. Now, dogs do not pass into cats.

I have seen, for instance, with a little overcrowding, continued fever grow up; and with a little more, typhoid fever; and with a little more, typhus, and all in the same ward or hut.

Would it not be far better, truer, and more practical, if we looked upon disease in this light?

For diseases, as all experience shows, are adjectives, not noun substantives.

[Original page no. 19]

not so even now, in some of the European lazarets—in which the plague-patient used to be condemned to the horrors of filth, over-crowding, and want of ventilation, while the medical attendant was ordered to examine the patient's tongue through an opera-glass and to toss him a lancet to open his abscesses with!

True nursing ignores infection, except to prevent it. Cleanliness and fresh air from open windows, with unremitting attention to the patient, are the only defence a true nurse either asks or needs.

Wise and humane management of the patient is the best safe-guard against infection.

Why must children have measles, &c. There are not a few popular opinions, in regard to which it is useful at times to ask a question or two. For example, it is com-monly thought that children must have what are commonly called "children's epidemics," "current contagions," &c., in other words, that they are born to have measles, hooping-cough, perhaps even scarlet fever, just as they are born to cut their teeth, if they live.

Now, do tell us, why must a child have measles?

Oh because, you say, we cannot keep it from infection—other children have measles—and it must take them—and it is safer that it should.

But why must other children have measles? And if they have, why must yours have them too?

If you believed in and observed the laws for preserving the health of houses which inculcate cleanliness, ventilation, white-washing, and other means, and which, by the way, *are laws*, as implicitly as you believe in the popular opinion, for it is nothing more than an opinion, that your child must have children's epidemics, don't you think that upon the whole your child would be more likely to escape altogether?

III. PETTY MANAGEMENT.

Petty management. All the results of good nursing, as detailed in these notes, may be spoiled or utterly negatived by one defect, viz.: in petty manage-ment, or, in other words, by not knowing how to manage that what you do when you are there, shall be done when you are not there. The most devoted friend or nurse cannot be always *there*. Nor is it desirable that she should. And she may give up her health, all her other duties, and yet, for want of a little management, be not one-half so efficient as another who is not one-half so devoted, but who has this art of multiplying herself—that is to say, the patient of the first will not really be so well cared for, as the patient of the second.

It is as impossible in a book to teach a person in charge of sick how to *manage*, as it is to teach her how to nurse. Circumstances must vary with each different case. But it *is* possible to press upon her to think for herself: Now what does happen during my absence? I am obliged to be away on Tuesday. But fresh air, or punctuality is not less important to my patient on Tuesday than it was on

Monday. Or: At 10 P.M. I am never with my patient; but quiet is of no less consequence to him at 10 than it was at 5 minutes to 10.

Curious as it may seem, this very obvious consideration occurs comparatively to few, or, if it does occur, it is only to cause the devoted friend or nurse to be absent fewer hours or fewer minutes from her patient—not to arrange so as that no minute and no hour shall be for her patient without the essentials of her nursing.

A very few instances will be sufficient, not as precepts, but as illustrations. *Illustrations of the want of it.*

A strange washerwoman, coming late at night for the "things," will burst in by mistake to the patient's sick-room, after he has fallen into his first doze, giving him a shock, the effects of which are irremediable, though he himself laughs at the cause, and probably never even mentions it. The nurse who is, and is quite right to be, at her supper, has not provided that the washerwoman shall not lose her way and go into the wrong room. *Strangers coming into the sick room.*

The patient's room may always have the window open. But the passage outside the patient's room, though provided with several large windows, may never have one open. Because it is not understood that the charge of the sick-room extends to the charge of the passage. And thus, as often happens, the nurse makes it her business to turn the patient's room into a ventilating shaft for the foul air of the whole house. *Sick room airing the whole house.*

An uninhabited room, a newly painted room,* an uncleaned closet or cupboard, may often become a reservoir of foul air for the whole house, because the person in charge never thinks of arranging that these places shall be always aired, always cleaned; she merely opens the window herself "when she goes in." *Uninhabited room fouling the whole house.*

An agitating letter or message may be delivered, or an important letter or message *not* delivered; a visitor whom it was of consequence to see, may be refused, or one whom it was of still more consequence *not* to see may be admitted—because the person in charge has never asked herself this question, What is done when I am not there? † *Delivery and non-delivery of letters and messages.*

At all events, one may safely say, a nurse cannot be with the

* That excellent paper, the *Builder*, mentions the lingering of the smell of paint for a month about a house as a proof of want of ventilation. Certainly— and, where there are ample windows to open, and these are never opened to get rid of the smell of paint, it is a proof of want of management in using the means of ventilation. Of course the smell will then remain for months. Why should it go? *Lingering smell of paint a want of care.*

† Why should you let your patient ever be surprised, except by thieves? I do not know. In England, people do not come down the chimney, or through the window, unless they are thieves. They come in by the door, and somebody must open the door to them. The "somebody" charged with opening the door is one of two, three, or at most four persons. Why cannot these, at most, four persons be put in charge as to what is to be done when there is a ring at the door bell? *Why let your patient ever be surprised*

The sentry at a post is changed much oftener than any servant at a private house or institution can possibly be. But what should we think of such an excuse as this: that the enemy had entered such a post because A and not B had been on guard? Yet I have constantly heard such an excuse made in the private house or institution and accepted: viz., that such a person had been "let in" or *not* "let in," and such a parcel had been wrongly delivered or lost because A and not B had opened the door!

[Original page no. 21]

patient, open the door, eat her meals, take a message, all at one and the same time. Nevertheless the person in charge never seems to look the impossibility in the face.

Add to this that the *attempting* this impossibility does more to increase the poor Patient's hurry and nervousness than anything else.

Partial measures such as "being always in the way" yourself, increase instead of saving the patient's anxiety. Because they must be only partial. It is never thought that the patient remembers these things if you do not. He has not only to think whether the visit or letter may arrive, but whether you will be in the way at the particular day and hour when it may arrive. So that your *partial* measures for "being in the way" yourself, only increase the necessity for his thought. Whereas, if you could but arrange that the thing should always be done whether you are there or not, he need never think at all about it.

For the above reasons, whatever a patient *can* do for himself, it is better, *i.e.* less anxiety, for him to do for himself, unless the person in charge has the spirit of management.

It is evidently much less exertion for a patient to answer a letter for himself by return of post, than to have four conversations, wait five days, have six anxieties before it is off his mind, before the person who is to answer it has done so.

Apprehension, uncertainty, waiting, expectation, fear of surprise, do a patient more harm than any exertion. Remember, he is face to face with his enemy all the time, internally wrestling with him, having long imaginary conversations with him. You are thinking of something else. "Rid him of his adversary quickly," is a first rule with the sick.*

For the same reasons, always tell a patient and tell him beforehand when you are going out and when you will be back, whether it is for a day, an hour, or ten minutes. You fancy perhaps that it is better for him if he does not find out your going at all, better for him if you do not make yourself "of too much importance" to him; or else you cannot bear to give him the pain or the anxiety of the temporary separation.

No such thing. You *ought* to go, we will suppose. Health or duty requires it. Then say so to the patient openly. If you go without his knowing it, and he finds it out, he never will feel secure again that the things which depend upon you will be done when you are away, and in nine cases out of ten he will be right. If you go out without telling him when you will be back, he can take no measures nor precautions as to the things which concern you both, or which you do for him.

What is the cause of half the accidents which happen? If you look into the reports of trials or accidents, and especially of suicides, or into the medical history of fatal cases, it is almost incredible how often the whole thing turns upon something which

---

* There are many physical operations where *cæteris paribus* the danger is in a direct ratio to the time the operation lasts; and *cæteris paribus* the operator's success will be in direct ratio to his quickness. Now there are many mental operations where exactly the same rule holds good with the sick; *cæteris paribus* their capability of bearing such operations depends directly on the quickness, *without hurry*, with which they can be got through.

has happened because "he," or still oftener "she," "was not there." But it is still more incredible how often, how almost always this is accepted as a sufficient reason, a justification; why, the very fact of the thing having happened is the proof of its not being a justification. The person in charge was quite right not to be "*there*," he was called away for quite sufficient reason, or he was away for a daily recurring and unavoidable cause: yet no provision was made to supply his absence. The fault was not in his "being away," but in there being no management to supplement his "being away." When the sun is under a total eclipse or during his nightly absence, we light candles. But it would seem as if it did not occur to us that we must also supplement the person in charge of sick or of children, whether under an occasional eclipse or during a regular absence.

In institutions where many lives would be lost and the effect of such want of management would be terrible and patent, there is less of it than in the private house.*

* So true is this that I could mention two cases of women of very high position, both of whom died in the same way of the consequences of a surgical operation. And in both cases, I was told by the highest authority that the fatal result would not have happened in a London hospital.

But, as far as regards the art of petty management in hospitals, all the military hospitals I know must be excluded. Upon my own experience I stand, and I solemnly declare that I have seen or known of fatal accidents, such as suicides in *delirium tremens*, bleedings to death, dying patients dragged out of bed by drunken Medical Staff Corps men, and many other things less patent and striking, which would not have happened in London civil hospitals nursed by women. The medical officers should be absolved from all blame in these accidents. How can a medical officer mount guard all day and all night over a patient (say) in *delirium tremens?* The fault lies in there being no organized system of attendance. Were a trustworthy *man* in charge of each ward, or set of wards, not as office clerk, but as head nurse, (and head nurse the best hospital serjeant, or ward master, is not now and cannot be, from default of the proper regulations), the thing would not, in all probability, have happened. But were a trustworthy *woman* in charge of the ward, or set of wards, the thing would not, in all certainty, have happened. In other words, it does not happen where a trustworthy woman is really in charge. And, in these remarks, I by no means refer only to exceptional times of great emergency in war hospitals, but also, and quite as much, to the ordinary run of military hospitals at home, in time of peace; or to a time in war when our army was actually more healthy than at home in peace, and the pressure on our hospitals consequently much less.

It is often said that, in regimental hospitals, patients ought to "nurse each other," because the number of sick altogether being, say, but thirty, and out of these one only perhaps being seriously ill, and the other twenty-nine having little the matter with them, and nothing to do, they should be set to nurse the one; also, that soldiers are so trained to obey, that they will be the most obedient, and therefore the best of nurses, add to which they are always kind to their comrades.

Now, have those who say this, considered that, in order to obey, you must know *how* to obey, and that these soldiers certainly do not know how to obey in nursing. I have seen these "kind" fellows (and how kind they are no one knows so well as myself) move a comrade so that, in one case at least, the man died in the act. I have seen the comrades' "kindness" produce abundance of spirits, to be drunk in secret. Let no one understand by this that female nurses ought to, or could be introduced in regimental hospitals. It would be most undesirable, even were it not impossible. But the head nurseship of a hospital

Petty management better understood in institutions than in private houses.

What institutions are the exception?

Nursing in Regimental Hospitals.

But in both, let whoever is in charge keep this simple question in her head (*not*, how can I always do this right thing myself, but) how can I provide for this right thing to be always done?

Then, when anything wrong has actually happened in consequence of her absence, which absence we will suppose to have been quite right, let her question still be (*not*, ｛how can I provide against any more of such absences? which is neither possible nor desirable, but) how can I provide against any thing wrong arising out of my absence?

What it is to be "in charge."

How few men, or even women, understand, either in great or in little things, what it is the being "in charge"—I mean, know how to carry out a "charge." From the most colossal calamities, down to the most trifling accidents, results are often traced (or rather *not* traced) to such want of some one "in charge" or of his knowing how to be "in charge." A short time ago the bursting of a funnel-casing on board the finest and strongest ship that ever was built, on her trial trip, destroyed several lives and put several hundreds in jeopardy—not from any undetected flaw in her new and untried works—but from a tap being closed which ought not to have been closed—from what every child knows would make its mother's tea-kettle burst. And this simply because no one seemed to know what it is to be "in charge," or *who* was in charge. Nay more, the jury at the inquest actually altogether ignored the same, and apparently considered the tap "in charge," for they gave as a verdict "accidental death."

This is the meaning of the word, on a large scale. On a much smaller scale, it happened, a short time ago, that an insane person burnt herself slowly and intentionally to death, while in her doctor's charge and almost in his nurse's presence. Yet neither was considered "at all to blame." The very fact of the accident happening proves its own case. There is nothing more to be said. Either they did not know their business or they did not know how to perform it.

To be "in charge" is certainly not only to carry out the proper measures yourself but to see that every one else does so too; to see that no one either wilfully or ignorantly thwarts or prevents such measures. It is neither to do everything yourself nor to appoint a number of people to each duty, but to ensure that each does that duty to which he is appointed. This is the meaning which must be attached to the word by (above all) those "in charge" of sick, whether of numbers or of individuals, (and indeed I think it is with individual sick that it is least understood. One sick person is often waited on by four with less precision, and is really less cared for than ten who are waited on by one; or at least than 40 who are waited on by 4; and all for want of this one person "in charge.)"

serjeant is the more essential, the more important, the more inexperienced the nurses. Undoubtedly, a London hospital "sister" does sometimes set relays of patients to watch a critical case; but, undoubtedly also, always under her own superintendence; and she is called to whenever there is something to be done, and she knows how to do it. The patients are not left to do it of their own unassisted genius, however "kind" and willing they may be.

It is often said that there are few good servants now: I say there are few good mistresses now. As the jury seems to have thought the tap was in charge of the ship's safety, so mistresses now seem to think the house is in charge of itself. They neither know how to give orders, nor how to teach their servants to obey orders—*i. e.* to obey intelligently, which is the real meaning of all discipline.

Again, people who are in charge often seem to have a pride in feeling that they will be "missed," that no one can understand or carry on their arrangements, their system, books, accounts, &c., but themselves. It seems to me that the pride is rather in carrying on a system, in keeping stores, closets, books, accounts, &c., so that any body can understand and carry them on—so that, in case of absence or illness, one can deliver every thing up to others and know that all will go on as usual, and that one shall never be missed.

NOTE.—It is often complained, that professional nurses, brought into private families, in case of sickness, make themselves intolerable by "ordering about" the other servants, under plea of not neglecting the patient. Both things are true; the patient is often neglected, and the servants are often unfairly "put upon." But the fault is generally in the want of management of the head in charge. It is surely for her to arrange both that the nurse's place is, when necessary, supplemented, and that the patient is never neglected—things with a little management quite compatible, and indeed only attainable together. It is certainly not for the nurse to "order about" the servants. *Why hired nurses give so much trouble.*

IV. NOISE.

Unnecessary noise, or noise that creates an expectation in the mind, is that which hurts a patient. It is rarely the loudness of the noise, the effect upon the organ of the ear itself, which appears to affect the sick. How well a patient will generally bear, *e.g.*, the putting up of a scaffolding close to the house, when he cannot bear the talking, still less the whispering, especially if it be of a familiar voice, outside his door. *Unnecessary noise.*

There are certain patients, no doubt, especially where there is slight concussion or other disturbance of the brain, who are affected by mere noise. But intermittent noise, or sudden and sharp noise, in these as in all other cases, affects far more than continuous noise—noise with jar far more than noise without. Of one thing you may be certain, that anything which wakes a patient suddenly out of his sleep will invariably put him into a state of greater excitement, do him more serious, aye, and lasting mischief, than any continuous noise, however loud.

Never to allow a patient to be waked, intentionally or accidentally, is a *sine quâ non* of all good nursing. If he is roused out of his first sleep, he is almost certain to have no more sleep. It is a curious but quite intelligible fact that, if a patient is waked after a few hours' instead of a few minutes' sleep, he is much more likely to sleep again. Because pain, like irritability of brain, perpetuates and intensifies itself. If you have gained a respite of either in sleep *Never let a patient be waked out of his first sleep.*

you have gained more than the mere respite. Both the probability
of recurrence and of the same intensity will be diminished; whereas
both will be terribly increased by want of sleep. This is the reason
why sleep is so all-important. This is the reason why a patient
waked in the early part of his sleep loses not only his sleep, but his
power to sleep. A healthy person who allows himself to sleep during
the day will lose his sleep at night. But it is exactly the reverse
with the sick generally; the more they sleep, the better will they
be able to sleep.

Noise which excites expectation.
I have often been surprised at the thoughtlessness, (resulting
in cruelty, quite unintentionally) of friends or of doctors who will
hold a long conversation just in the room or passage adjoining to
the room of the patient, who is either every moment expecting
them to come in, or who has just seen them, and knows they are
talking about him. If he is an amiable patient, he will try to
occupy his attention elsewhere and not to listen—and this makes
matters worse—for the strain upon his attention and the effort he
makes are so great that it is well if he is not worse for hours

Whispered conversation in the room.
after. If it is a whispered conversation in the same room, then
it is absolutely cruel; for it is impossible that the patient's attention
should not be involuntarily strained to hear. Walking on tip-toe,
doing any thing in the room very slowly, are injurious, for exactly the
same reasons. A firm light quick step, a steady quick hand are the
desiderata; not the slow, lingering, shuffling foot, the timid, uncertain
touch. Slowness is not gentleness, though it is often mistaken for
such; quickness, lightness, and gentleness are quite compatible.
Again, if friends and doctors did but watch, as nurses can and
should watch, the features sharpening, the eyes growing almost wild,
of fever patients who are listening for the entrance from the
corridor of the persons whose voices they are hearing there, these
would never run the risk again of creating such expectation, or
irritation of mind.—Such unnecessary noise has undoubtedly induced
or aggravated delirium in many cases. I have known such—in one
case death ensued. It is but fair to say that this death was attributed to fright. It was the result of a long whispered conversation,
within sight of the patient, about an impending operation; but any
one who has known the more than stoicism, the cheerful coolness, with
which the certainty of an operation will be accepted by any patient,
capable of bearing an operation at all, if it is properly communicated to him, will hesitate to believe that it was mere fear which produced, as was averred, the fatal result in this instance. It was rather
the uncertainty, the strained expectation as to what was to be decided
upon.

Or just out-side the door.
I need hardly say that the other common cause, namely, for a
doctor or friend to leave the patient and communicate his opinion
on the result of his visit to the friends just outside the patient's door,
or in the adjoining room, after the visit, but within hearing or knowledge of the patient is, if possible, worst of all.

Noise of female dress.
It is, I think, alarming, peculiarly at this time, when the female
ink-bottles are perpetually impressing upon us "woman's" "parti-

cular worth and general missionariness," to see that the dress of women is daily more and more unfitting them for any "mission," or usefulness at all. It is equally unfitted for all poetic and all domestic purposes. A man is now a more handy and far less objectionable being in a sick-room than a woman. Compelled by her dress, every woman now either shuffles or waddles—only a man can cross the floor of a sick-room without shaking it! What is become of woman's light step?—the firm, light, quick step we have been asking for?

Unnecessary noise, then, is the most cruel absence of care which can be inflicted either on sick or well. For, in all these remarks, the sick are only mentioned as suffering in a greater proportion than the well from precisely the same causes.

Unnecessary (although slight) noise injures a sick person much more than necessary noise (of a much greater amount).

All doctrines about mysterious affinities and aversions will be found to resolve themselves very much, if not entirely, into presence or absence of care in these things. Patient's repulsion to nurses who rustle.

A nurse who rustles (I am speaking of nurses professional and unprofessional) is the horror of a patient, though perhaps he does not know why.

The fidget of silk and of crinoline, the rattling of keys, the creaking of stays and of shoes, will do a patient more harm than all the medicines in the world will do him good.

The noiseless step of woman, the noiseless drapery of woman, are mere figures of speech in this day. Her skirts (and well if they do not throw down some piece of furniture) will at least brush against every article in the room as she moves.*

Again, one nurse cannot open the door without making everything rattle. Or she opens the door unnecessarily often, for want of remembering all the articles that might be brought in at once.

A good nurse will always make sure that no door or window in her patient's room shall rattle or creak; that no blind or curtain shall, by any change of wind through the open window, be made to flap—especially will she be careful of all this before she leaves her patients for the night. If you wait till your patients tell you, or remind you of these things, where is the use of their having a nurse? There are more shy than exacting patients, in all classes; and many

---

* Fortunate it is if her skirts do not catch fire—and if the nurse does not give Burning of the crinolines. herself up a sacrifice together with her patient, to be burnt in her own petticoats. I wish the Registrar-General would tell us the exact number of deaths by burning occasioned by this absurd and hideous custom. But if people will be stupid, let them take measures to protect themselves from their own stupidity—measures which every chemist knows, such as putting alum into starch, which prevents starched articles of dress from blazing up.

I wish too that people who wear crinoline could see the indecency of their Indecency of the crinolines. own dress as other people see it. A respectable elderly woman stooping forward, invested in crinoline, exposes quite as much of her own person to the patient lying in the room as any opera dancer does on the stage. But no one will ever tell her this unpleasant truth.

a patient passes a bad night, time after time, rather than remind his nurse every night of all the things she has forgotten.

If there are blinds to your windows, always take care to have them well up, when they are not being used. A little piece slipping down, and flapping with every draught, will distract a patient.

Hurry peculiarly hurtful to sick.

All hurry or bustle is peculiarly painful to the sick. And when a patient has compulsory occupations to engage him, instead of having simply to amuse himself, it becomes doubly injurious. The friend who remains standing and fidgetting about while a patient is talking business to him, or the friend who sits and proses, the one from an idea of not letting the patient talk, the other from an idea of amusing him,—each is equally inconsiderate. Always sit down when a sick person is talking business to you, show no signs of hurry, give complete attention and full consideration if your advice is wanted, and go away the moment the subject is ended.

How to visit the sick and not hurt them.

Always sit within the patient's view, so that when you speak to him he has not painfully to turn his head round in order to look at you. Everybody involuntarily looks at the person speaking. If you make this act a wearisome one on the part of the patient you are doing him harm. So also if by continuing to stand you make him continuously raise his eyes to see you. Be as motionless as possible, and never gesticulate in speaking to the sick.

Never make a patient repeat a message or request, especially if it be some time after. Occupied patients are often accused of doing too much of their own business. They are instinctively right. How often you hear the person, charged with the request of giving the message or writing the letter, say half an hour afterwards to the patient, "Did you appoint 12 o'clock?" or, "What did you say was the address?" or ask perhaps some much more agitating question—thus causing the patient the effort of memory, or worse still, of decision, all over again. It is really less exertion to him to write his letters himself. This is the almost universal experience of occupied invalids.

This brings us to another caution. Never speak to an invalid from behind, nor from the door, nor from any distance from him, nor when he is doing anything.

The official politeness of servants in these things is so grateful to invalids, that many prefer, without knowing why, having none but servants about them.

These things not fancy.

These things are not fancy. If we consider that, with sick as with well, every thought decomposes some nervous matter,—that decomposition as well as re-composition of nervous matter is always going on, and more quickly with the sick than with the well,—that, to obtrude abruptly another thought upon the brain while it is in the act of destroying nervous matter by thinking, is calling upon it to make a new exertion,—if we consider these things, which are facts, not fancies, we shall remember that we are doing positive injury by interrupting, by "startling a fanciful" person, as it is

Interruption damaging to sick.

called. Alas! it is no fancy.

If the invalid is forced, by his avocations, to continue occupations

[Original page no. 28]

requiring much thinking, the injury is doubly great. In feeding a patient suffering under delirium or stupor you may suffocate him, by giving him his food suddenly, but if you rub his lips gently with a spoon and thus attract his attention, he will swallow the food unconsciously, but with perfect safety. Thus it is with the brain. If you offer it a thought, especially one requiring a decision, abruptly, you do it a real not fanciful injury. Never speak to a sick person suddenly; but, at the same time, do not keep his expectation on the tiptoe.

This rule, indeed, applies to the well quite as much as to the sick. And to well. I have never known persons who exposed themselves for years to constant interruption who did not muddle away their intellects by it at last. The process with them may be accomplished without pain. With the sick, pain gives warning of the injury.

Do not meet or overtake a patient who is moving about in order Keeping a to speak to him, or to give him any message or letter. You might patient just as well give him a box on the ear. I have seen a patient fall standing. flat on the ground who was standing when his nurse came into the room. This was an accident which might have happened to the most careful nurse. But the other is done with intention. A patient in such a state is not going to the East Indies. If you would wait ten seconds, or walk ten yards further, any promenade he could make would be over. You do not know the effort it is to a patient to remain standing for even a quarter of a minute to listen to you. If I had not seen the thing done by the kindest nurses and friends, I should have thought this caution quite superfluous.*

Patients are often accused of being able to "do much more when Patients dread nobody is by." It is quite true that they can. Unless nurses can surprise. be brought to attend to considerations of the kind of which we have given here but a few specimens, a very weak patient finds it really much less exertion to do things for himself than to ask for them. And he will, in order to do them, (very innocently and from instinct) calculate the time his nurse is likely to be absent, from a fear of her "coming in upon" him or speaking to him, just at the moment when he finds it quite as much as he can do to crawl from his bed to his chair, or from one room to another, or down stairs, or out of doors for a few minutes. Some extra call made upon his attention at that moment will quite upset him. In these cases you may be sure that a patient in the state we have described does not make such exertions more than once or twice a-day, and probably

---

* It is absolutely essential that a nurse should lay this down as a positive rule Never speak to to herself, never to speak to any patient who is standing or moving, as long as a patient in she exercises so little observation as not to know when a patient cannot bear it. the act of I am satisfied that many of the accidents which happen from feeble patients tumb- moving. ling down stairs, fainting after getting up, &c., happen solely from the nurse popping out of a door to speak to the patient just at that moment; or from his fearing that she will do so. And that if the patient were even left to himself, till he can sit down, such accidents would much seldomer occur. If the nurse accompanies the patient let her not call upon him to speak. It is incredible that nurses cannot picture to themselves the strain upon the heart, the lungs, and the brain which the act of moving is to any feeble patient.

[Original page no. 29]

much about the same hour every day. And it is hard, indeed, if nurse and friends cannot calculate so as to let him make them undisturbed. Remember, that many patients can walk who cannot stand or even sit up. Standing is, of all positions, the most trying to a weak patient.

Everything you do in a patient's room, after he is "put up" for the night, increases tenfold the risk of his having a bad night. But, if you rouse him up after he has fallen asleep, you do not risk, you secure him a bad night.

One hint I would give to all who attend or visit the sick, to all who have to pronounce an opinion upon sickness or its progress. Come back and look at your patient *after* he has had an hour's animated conversation with you. It is the best test of his real state we know. But never pronounce upon him from merely seeing what he does, or how he looks, during such a conversation. Learn also carefully and exactly, if you can, how he passed the night after it.

Effects of over-exertion on sick.

People rarely, if ever, faint while making an exertion. It is after it is over. Indeed, almost every effect of over-exertion appears after, not during such exertion. It is the highest folly to judge of the sick, as is so often done, when you see them merely during a period of excitement. People have very often died of that which, it has been proclaimed at the time, has "done them no harm."*

Remember never to lean against, sit upon, or unnecessarily shake, or even touch the bed in which a patient lies. This is invariably a painful annoyance. If you shake the chair on which he sits, he has a point by which to steady himself, in his feet. But on a bed or sofa, he is entirely at your mercy, and he feels every jar you give him all through him.

Difference between real and fancy patients.

In all that we have said, both here and elsewhere, let it be distinctly understood that we are not speaking of hypochondriacs. To distinguish between real and fancied disease forms an important branch of the education of a nurse. To manage fancy patients forms an important branch of her duties. But the nursing which real and that which fancied patients require is of different, or rather of opposite, character. And the latter will not be spoken of here. Indeed, many of the symptoms which are here mentioned are those which distinguish real from fancied disease.

Careless observation of the results of careless visits.

* As an old experienced nurse, I do most earnestly deprecate all such careless words. I have known patients delirious all night, after seeing a visitor who called them "better," thought they "only wanted a little amusement," and who came again, saying, "I hope you were not the worse for my visit," neither waiting for an answer, nor even looking at the case. No real patient will ever say, "Yes, but I was a great deal the worse."

It is not, however, either death or delirium of which, in these cases, there is most danger to the patient. Unperceived consequences are far more likely to ensue. *You* will have impunity—the poor patient will *not*. That is, the patient will suffer, although neither he nor the inflictor of the injury will attribute it to its real cause. It will not be directly traceable, except by a very careful observant nurse. The patient will often not even mention what has done him most harm.

It is true that hypochondriacs very often do that behind a nurse's back which they would not do before her face. Many such I have had as patients who scarcely ate anything at their regular meals; but if you concealed food for them in a drawer, they would take it at night or in secret. But this is from quite a different motive. They do it from the wish to conceal. Whereas the real patient will often boast to his nurse or doctor, if these do not shake their heads at him, of how much he has done, or eaten, or walked. To return to real disease.

Conciseness and decision are, above all things, necessary with the sick. Let your thought expressed to them be concisely and decidedly expressed. What doubt and hesitation there may be in your own mind must never be communicated to theirs, not even (I would rather say especially not) in little things. Let your doubt be to yourself, your decision to them. People who think outside their heads, the whole process of whose thought appears, like Homer's, in the act of secretion, who tell everything that led them towards this conclusion and away from that, ought never to be with the sick.

Conciseness necessary with Sick.

Irresolution is what all patients most dread. Rather than meet this in others, they will collect all their data, and make up their minds for themselves. A change of mind in others, whether it is regarding an operation, or re-writing a letter, always injures the patient more than the being called upon to make up his mind to the most dreaded or difficult decision. Farther than this, in very many cases, the imagination in disease is far more active and vivid than it is in health. If you propose to the patient change of air to one place one hour, and to another the next, he has, in each case, immediately constituted himself in imagination the tenant of the place, gone over the whole premises in idea, and you have tired him as much by displacing his imagination, as if you had actually carried him over both places.

Irresolution most painful to them.

Above all leave the sick room quickly and come into it quickly, not suddenly, not with a rush. But don't let the patient be wearily waiting for when you will be out of the room or when you will be in it. Conciseness and decision in your movements, as well as your words, are necessary in the sick room, as necessary as absence of hurry and bustle. To possess yourself entirely will ensure you from either failing—either loitering or hurrying.

If a patient has to see, not only to his own but also to his nurse's punctuality, or perseverance, or readiness, or calmness, to any or all of these things, he is far better without that nurse than with her— however valuable and handy her services may otherwise be to him, and however incapable he may be of rendering them to himself.

What a patient must not have to see to.

With regard to reading aloud in the sick room, my experience is, that when the sick are too ill to read to themselves, they can seldom bear to be read to. Children, eye-patients, and uneducated persons are exceptions, or where there is any mechanical difficulty in reading. People who like to be read to, have generally not much the matter with them; while in fevers, or where there is much irritability of brain, the effort of listening to reading aloud has often

Reading aloud.

brought on delirium. I speak with great diffidence; because there is an almost universal impression that it is *sparing* the sick to read aloud to them. But two things are certain:—

Read aloud slowly, distinctly, and steadily to the sick.

(1.) If there is some matter which *must* be read to a sick person, do it slowly. People often think that the way to get it over with least fatigue to him is to get it over in least time. They gabble; they plunge and gallop through the reading. There never was a greater mistake. Houdin, the conjuror, says that the way to make a story seem short is to tell it slowly. So it is with reading to the sick. I have often heard a patient say to such a mistaken reader, "Don't read it to me; tell it me."* Unconsciously he is aware that this will regulate the plunging, the reading with unequal paces, slurring over one part, instead of leaving it out altogether, if it is unimportant, and mumbling another. If the reader lets his own attention wander, and then stops to read up to himself, or finds he has read the wrong bit, then it is all over with the poor patient's chance of not suffering. Very few people know how to read to the sick; very few read aloud as pleasantly even as they speak. In reading they sing, they hesitate, they stammer, they hurry, they mumble; when in speaking they do none of these things. Reading aloud to the sick ought always to be rather slow, and exceedingly distinct, but not mouthing—rather monotonous, but not sing song—rather loud, but not noisy—and, above all, not too long. Be very sure of what your patient can bear.

Never read aloud by fits and starts to the sick.

(2.) The extraordinary habit of reading to oneself in a sick room, and reading aloud to the patient any bits which will amuse him or more often the reader, is unaccountably thoughtless. What *do* you think the patient is thinking of during your gaps of non-reading? Do you think that he amuses himself upon what you have read for precisely the time it pleases you to go on reading to yourself, and that his attention is ready for something else at precisely the time it pleases you to begin reading again? Whether the person thus read to be sick or well, whether he be doing nothing or doing something else while being thus read to, the self-absorption and want of observation of the person who does it, is equally difficult to understand—although very often the read*ee* is too amiable to say how much it disturbs him.

People overhead.

One thing more:—From the flimsy manner in which most modern houses are built, where every step on the stairs, and along the floors, is felt all over the house; the higher the story, the greater the vibration. It is inconceivable how much the sick suffer by having anybody overhead. In the solidly built old houses, which, fortunately, most hospitals are, the noise and shaking is comparatively trifling. But it is a serious cause of suffering, in lightly built houses, and with the irritability peculiar to some diseases. Better far put such patients at the top of the house, even with the additional fatigue of stairs, if you cannot secure the room above them being

The sick would rather be told a thing than have it read to them.

* Sick children, if not too shy to speak, will always express this wish. They invariably prefer a story to be *told* to them, rather than read to them.

untenanted; you may otherwise bring on a state of restlessness which no opium will subdue. Do not neglect the warning, when a patient tells you that he " Feels every step above him to cross his heart." Remember that every noise a patient cannot *see* partakes of the character of suddenness to him; and I am persuaded that patients with these peculiarly irritable nerves, are positively less injured by having persons in the same room with them than overhead, or separated by only a thin compartment. Any sacrifice to secure silence for these cases is worth while, because no air, however good, no attendance, however careful, will do anything for such cases without quiet.

NOTE.—The effect of music upon the sick has been scarcely at all noticed. In fact, its expensiveness, as it is now, makes any general application of it quite out of the question. I will only remark here, that wind instruments, including the human voice, and stringed instruments, capable of continuous sound, have generally a beneficent effect—while the piano-forte, with such instruments as have *no* continuity of sound, has just the reverse. The finest piano-forte playing will damage the sick, while an air, like " Home, sweet home," or " Assisa a piè d'un salice," on the most ordinary grinding organ will sensibly soothe them—and this quite independent of association. — Music.

V. VARIETY.

To any but an old nurse, or an old patient, the degree would be quite inconceivable to which the nerves of the sick suffer from seeing the same walls, the same ceiling, the same surroundings during a long confinement to one or two rooms. — Variety a means of recovery.

The superior cheerfulness of persons suffering severe paroxysms of pain over that of persons suffering from nervous debility has often been remarked upon, and attributed to the enjoyment of the former of their intervals of respite. I incline to think that the majority of cheerful cases is to be found among those patients who are not confined to one room, whatever their suffering, and that the majority of depressed cases will be seen among those subjected to a long monotony of objects about them.

The nervous frame really suffers as much from this as the digestive organs from long monotony of diet, as *e.g.* the soldier from his twenty-one years' " boiled beef."

The effect in sickness of beautiful objects, of variety of objects, and especially of brilliancy of colour is hardly at all appreciated. — Colour and form means of recovery.

Such cravings are usually called the "fancies" of patients. And often doubtless patients have "fancies," as, *e.g.* when they desire two contradictions. But much more often, their (so called)"fancies" are the most valuable indications of what is necessary for their recovery. And it would be well if nurses would watch these (so called) "fancies" closely.

I have seen, in fevers (and felt, when I was a fever patient myself) the most acute suffering produced from the patient (in a hut) not being able to see out of window, and the knots in the wood being the only view. I shall never forget the rapture of fever patients over a bunch of bright-coloured flowers. I remember (in my own case) a nosegay of wild flowers being sent me, and from that moment recovery becoming more rapid.

This is no fancy.

People say the effect is only on the mind. It is no such thing. The effect is on the body, too. Little as we know about the way in which we are affected by form, by colour, and light, we do know this, that they have an actual physical effect.

Variety of form and brilliancy of colour in the objects presented to patients are actual means of recovery.

But it must be *slow* variety, e. g., if you shew a patient ten or twelve engravings successively, ten-to-one that he does not become cold and faint, or feverish, or even sick; but hang one up opposite him, one on each successive day, or week, or month, and he will revel in the variety.

Flowers.

The folly and ignorance which reign too often supreme over the sick-room, cannot be better exemplified than by this. While the nurse will leave the patient stewing in a corrupting atmosphere, the best ingredient of which is carbonic acid; she will deny him, on the plea of unhealthiness, a glass of cut-flowers, or a growing plant. Now, no one ever saw "overcrowding" by plants in a room or ward. And the carbonic acid they give off at nights would not poison a fly. Nay, in overcrowded rooms, they actually absorb carbonic acid and give off oxygen. Cut-flowers also decompose water and produce oxygen gas. It is true there are certain flowers, e.g., lilies, the smell of which is said to depress the nervous system. These are easily known by the smell, and can be avoided.

Effect of body on mind.

Volumes are now written and spoken upon the effect of the mind upon the body. Much of it is true. But I wish a little more was thought of the effect of the body on the mind. You who believe yourselves overwhelmed with anxieties, but are able every day to walk up Regent-street, or out in the country, to take your meals with others in other rooms, &c., &c., you little know how much your anxieties are thereby lightened; you little know how intensified they become to those who can have no change;* how the very walls of their sick rooms seem hung with their cares; how the ghosts of their troubles haunt their beds; how impossible it is for them to escape from a pursuing thought without some help from variety.

A patient can just as much move his leg when it is fractured as change his thoughts when no external help from variety is given him. This is, indeed, one of the main sufferings of sickness; just

Sick suffer to excess from mental as well as bodily pain.

* It is a matter of painful wonder to the sick themselves how much painful ideas predominate over pleasurable ones in their impressions; they reason with themselves; they think themselves ungrateful; it is all of no use. The fact is, that these painful impressions are far better dismissed by a real laugh, if you can excite one by books or conversation, than by any direct reasoning; or if the patient is too weak to laugh, some impression from nature is what he wants. I have mentioned the cruelty of letting him stare at a dead wall. In many diseases, especially in convalescence from fever, that wall will appear to make all sorts of faces at him; now flowers never do this. Form, colour, will free your patient from his painful ideas better than any argument.

as the fixed posture is one of the main sufferings of the broken limb.

It is an ever recurring wonder to see educated people, who call themselves nurses, acting thus. They vary their own objects, their own employments, many times a day; and while nursing (!) some bed-ridden sufferer, they let him lie there staring at a dead wall, without any change of object to enable him to vary his thoughts; and it never even occurs to them, at least to move his bed so that he can look out of window. No, the bed is to be always left in the darkest, dullest, remotest, part of the room.* {Help the sick to vary their thoughts.}

I think it is a very common error among the well to think that "with a little more self-control" the sick might, if they choose, "dismiss painful thoughts" which "aggravate their disease," &c. Believe me, almost *any* sick person, who behaves decently well, exercises more self-control every moment of his day than you will ever know till you are sick yourself. Almost every step that crosses his room is painful to him; almost every thought that crosses his brain is painful to him; and if he can speak without being savage, and look without being unpleasant, he is exercising self-control.

Suppose you have been up all night, and instead of being allowed to have your cup of tea, you were to be told that you ought to "exercise self-control," what should you say? Now, the nerves of the sick are always in the state that yours are in after you have been up all night.

We will suppose the diet of the sick to be cared for. Then, this state of nerves is most frequently to be relieved by care in affording them a pleasant view, a judicious variety as to flowers,† and pretty things. Light by itself will often relieve it. The craving for "the return of day," which the sick so constantly evince, is generally nothing but the desire for light, the remembrance of the relief which a variety of objects before the eye affords to the harassed sick mind. {Supply to the sick the defect of manual labour.}

Again, every man and every woman has some amount of manual employment; excepting a few fine ladies, who do not even dress themselves, and who are virtually in the same category, as to nerves, as the sick. Now, you can have no idea of the relief which manual labour is to you—of the degree to which the deprivation of manual

---

* I remember a case in point. A man received an injury to the spine, from an accident, which after a long confinement ended in death. He was a workman —had not in his composition a single grain of what is called "enthusiasm for nature."—but he was desperate to "see once more out of window." His nurse actually got him on her back, and managed to perch him up at the window for an instant, "to see out." The consequence to the poor nurse was a serious illness, which nearly proved fatal. The man never knew it; but a great many other people did. Yet the consequence in none of their minds, so far as I know, was the conviction that the craving for variety in the starving eye, is just as desperate as that for food in the starving stomach, and tempts the famishing creature in either case to steal for its satisfaction. No other word will express it but "desperation." And it sets the seal of ignorance and stupidity just as much on the governors and attendants of the sick, if they do not provide the sick-bed with a "view" of some kind, as if they did not provide the hospital with a kitchen. {Desperate desire in the sick to "see out of window."}

† No one who has watched the sick can doubt the fact, that some feel stimulus from looking at scarlet flowers, exhaustion from looking at deep blue, &c. {Physical effect of colour.}

employment increases the peculiar irritability from which many sick suffer.

A little needle-work, a little writing, a little cleaning, would be the greatest relief the sick could have, if they could do it; these *are* the greatest relief to you, though you do not know it. Reading, though it is often the only thing the sick can do, is not this relief. Bearing this in mind, bearing in mind that you have all these varieties of employment which the sick cannot have, bear also in mind to obtain for them all the varieties which they can enjoy.

I need hardly say that I am well aware that excess in needle-work, in writing, in any other continuous employment, will produce the same irritability that defect in manual employment (as one cause) produces in the sick.

VI. TAKING FOOD.

Want of attention to hours of taking food. Every careful observer of the sick will agree in this that thousands of patients are annually starved in the midst of plenty, from want of attention to the ways which alone make it possible for them to take food. This want of attention is as remarkable in those who urge upon the sick to do what is quite impossible to them, as in the sick themselves who will not make the effort to do what is perfectly possible to them.

For instance, to the large majority of very weak patients it is quite impossible to take any solid food before 11 A.M., nor then, if their strength is still further exhausted by fasting till that hour. For weak patients have generally feverish nights and, in the morning, dry mouths; and, if they could eat with those dry mouths, it would be the worse for them. A spoonful of beef-tea, of arrowroot and wine, of egg flip, every hour, will give them the requisite nourishment, and prevent them from being too much exhausted to take at a later hour the solid food, which is necessary for their recovery. And every patient who can swallow at all can swallow these liquid things, if he chooses. But how often do we hear a mutton-chop, an egg, a bit of bacon, ordered to a patient for breakfast, to whom (as a moment's consideration would show us) it must be quite impossible to masticate such things at that hour.

Again, a nurse is ordered to give a patient a tea-cup full of some article of food every three hours. The patient's stomach rejects it. If so, try a table-spoon full every hour; if this will not do, a tea-spoon full every quarter of an hour.

I am bound to say, that I think more patients are lost by want of care and ingenuity in these momentous minutiæ in private nursing than in public hospitals. And I think there is more of the *entente cordiale* to assist one another's hands between the doctor and his head nurse in the latter institutions, than between the doctor and the patient's friends in the private house.

Life often hangs upon minutes in taking food. If we did but know the consequences which may ensue, in very weak patients, from ten minutes' fasting or repletion, (I call it repletion when they are obliged to let too small an interval elapse between taking food and some other exertion, owing to the nurse's unpunctuality), we should be more careful never to let this occur. In very weak patients there is often a nervous difficulty of swallowing, which is so much increased by any other call upon their strength that, unless they have their food punctually at the minute, which minute again must be arranged so as to fall in with no other minute's occupation, they can take nothing till the next respite occurs—so that an unpunctuality or delay of ten minutes may very well turn out to be one of two or three hours. And why is it not as easy to be punctual to a minute? Life often literally hangs upon these minutes.

In acute cases, where life or death is to be determined in a few hours, these matters are very generally attended to, especially in Hospitals ; and the number of cases is large where the patient is, as it were, brought back to life by exceeding care on the part of the Doctor or Nurse, or both, in ordering and giving nourishment with minute selection and punctuality.

But, in chronic cases, lasting over months and years, where the fatal issue is often determined at last by mere protracted starvation, I had rather not enumerate the instances which I have known where a little ingenuity, and a great deal of perseverance, might, in all probability, have averted the result. The consulting the hours when the patient can take food, the observation of the times, often varying, when he is most faint, the altering seasons of taking food, in order to anticipate and prevent such times—all this, which requires observation, ingenuity, and perseverance (and these really constitute the good Nurse), might save more lives than we wot of. *Patients often starved to death in chronic cases.*

To leave the patient's untasted food by his side, from meal to meal, in hopes that he will eat it in the interval, is simply to prevent him from taking any food at all. I have known patients literally incapacitated from taking one article of food after another, by this piece of ignorance. Let the food come at the right time, and be taken away, eaten or uneaten, at the right time; but never let a patient have "something always standing" by him, if you don't wish to disgust him of everything. *Food never to be left by the patient's side.*

On the other hand, I have known a patient's life saved (he was sinking for want of food) by the simple question, put to him by the doctor, " But is there no hour when you feel you could eat? " " Oh, yes," he said, " I could always take something at — o'clock and — o'clock." The thing was tried and succeeded. Patients very seldom, however, can tell this ; it is for you to watch and find it out.

A patient should, if possible, not see or smell either the food of others, or a greater amount of food than he himself can consume at one time, or even hear food talked about or see it in the raw state. I know of no exception to the above rule. The breaking of it always induces a greater or less incapacity of taking food. *Patient had better not see more food than his own.*

In hospital wards it is of course impossible to observe all this ; and in single wards, where a patient must be continuously and closely watched, it is frequently impossible to relieve the attendant, so that his or her own meals can be taken out of the ward. But it is not the less true that, in such cases, even where the patient is not himself aware of it, his possibility of taking food is limited by seeing the attendant eating meals under his observation. In some cases the sick are aware of it, and complain. A case where the patient was supposed to be insensible, but complained as soon as able to speak, is now present to my recollection.

Remember, however, that the extreme punctuality in well-ordered hospitals, the rule that nothing shall be done in the ward while the patients are having their meals, go far to counterbalance what unavoidable evil there is in having patients together. I have often seen the private nurse go on dusting or fidgeting about in a sick room all the while the patient is eating, or trying to eat.

That the more alone an invalid can be when taking food, the better, is unquestionable; and, even if he must be fed, the nurse should not allow him to talk, or talk to him, especially about food, while eating.

When a person is compelled, by the pressure of occupation, to continue his business while sick, it ought to be a rule WITHOUT ANY EXCEPTION WHATEVER, that no one shall bring business to him or talk to him while he is taking food, nor go on talking to him on interesting subjects up to the last moment before his meals, nor make an engagement with him immediately after, so that there be any hurry of mind while taking them.

Upon the observance of these rules, especially the first, often depends the patient's capability of taking food at all, or, if he is amiable and forces himself to take food, of deriving any nourishment from it.

You cannot be too careful as to quality in sick diet. A nurse should never put before a patient milk that is sour, meat or soup that is turned, an egg that is bad, or vegetables underdone. Yet often I have seen these things brought in to the sick in a state perfectly perceptible to every nose or eye except the nurse's. It is here that the clever nurse appears; she will not bring in the peccant article, but, not to disappoint the patient, she will whip up something else in a few minutes. Remember that sick cookery should half do the work of your poor patient's weak digestion. But if you further impair it with your bad articles, I know not what is to become of him or of it.

If the nurse is an intelligent being, and not a mere carrier of diets to and from the patient, let her exercise her intelligence in these things. How often we have known a patient eat nothing at all in the day, because one meal was left untasted (at that time he was incapable of eating), at another the milk was sour, the third was spoiled by some other accident. And it never occurred to the nurse to extemporize some expedient,—it never occurred to her that as he had had no solid food that day, he might eat a bit of toast (say) with his tea in the evening, or he might have some meal an hour earlier. A patient who cannot touch his dinner at two, will often accept it gladly, if brought to him at seven. But somehow nurses never "think of these things." One would imagine they did not consider themselves bound to exercise their judgment; they leave it to the patient. Now I am quite sure that it is better for a patient rather, to suffer these neglects than to try to teach his nurse to nurse him, if she does not know how. It ruffles him, and if he is ill he is in no condition to teach, especially upon himself. The above remarks apply much more to private nursing than to hospitals.

I would say to the nurse, have a rule of thought about your patient's diet; consider, remember how much he has had, and how much he ought to have to-day. Generally, the only rule of the private patient's diet is what the nurse has to give. It is true she cannot give him what she has not got; but his stomach does not wait for her convenience, or even her necessity.* If it is used to having its stimulus at one hour to-day, and to-morrow it does not have it, because she has failed in getting it, he will suffer. She must be always exercising her ingenuity to supply defects, and to remedy accidents which will happen among the best contrivers, but from which the patient does not suffer the less, because "they cannot be helped." *[Nurse must have some rule of thought about her patient's diet.]*

One very minute caution,—take care not to spill into your patient's saucer, in other words, take care that the outside bottom rim of his cup shall be quite dry and clean; if, every time he lifts his cup to his lips, he has to carry the saucer with it, or else to drop the liquid upon, and to soil his sheet, or his bed-gown, or pillow, or if he is sitting up, his dress, you have no idea what a difference this minute want of care on your part makes to his comfort and even to his willingness for food *[Keep your patient's cup dry underneath.]*

VII. WHAT FOOD?

I will mention one or two of the most common errors among women in charge of sick respecting sick diet. One is the belief that beef tea is the most nutritive of all articles. Now, just try and boil down a lb. of beef into beef tea, evaporate your beef tea, and see what is left of your beef. You will find that there is barely a tea-spoonful of solid nourishment to half a pint of water in beef tea;—nevertheless there is a certain reparative quality in it, we do not know what, as there is in tea;—but it may safely be given in almost any inflammatory disease, and is as little to be depended upon with the healthy or convalescent where much nourishment is required. Again, it is an ever ready saw that an egg is equivalent to a lb. of meat,—whereas it is not at all so. Also, it is seldom noticed with how many *[Common errors in diet.]* *[Beef tea.]*

* Why, because the nurse has not got some food to-day which the patient takes, can the patient wait four hours for food to-day, who could not wait two hours yesterday? Yet this is the only logic one generally hears. On the other hand, the other logic, viz., of the nurse giving a patient a thing because she *has* got it, is equally fatal. If she happens to have fresh jelly, or fresh fruit, she will frequently give it to the patient half-an-hour after his dinner, or at his dinner, when he cannot possibly eat that and the broth too—or worse still leave it by his bed-side till he is so sickened with the sight of it, that he cannot eat it at all. *[Nurse must have some rule of time about the patient's diet.]*

Eggs.

patients, particularly of nervous or bilious temperament, eggs disagree. All puddings made with eggs, are distasteful to them in consequence. An egg, whipped up with wine, is often the only form in which they can take this kind of nourishment. Again, if the patient has attained to eating meat, it is supposed that to give him meat is the

Meat without vegetables.

only thing needful for his recovery; whereas scorbutic sores have been actually known to appear among sick persons living in the midst of plenty in England, which could be traced to no other source than this, viz.: that the nurse, depending on meat alone, had allowed the patient to be without vegetables for a considerable time, these latter being so badly cooked that he always left them untouched.

Arrowroot.

Arrowroot is another grand dependence of the nurse. As a vehicle for wine, and as a restorative quickly prepared, it is all very well. But it is nothing but starch and water. Flour is both more nutritive, and less liable to ferment, and is preferable wherever it can be used.

Milk, butter, cream, &c.

Again, milk and the preparations from milk, are a most important article of food for the sick. Butter is the lightest kind of animal fat, and though it wants the sugar and some of the other elements which there are in milk, yet it is most valuable both in itself and in enabling the patient to eat more bread. Flour, oats, groats, barley, and their kind, are as we have already said, preferable in all their preparations to all the preparations of arrow root, sago, tapioca, and their kind. Cream, in many long chronic diseases, is quite irreplaceable by any other article whatever. It seems to act in the same manner as beef tea, and to most it is much easier of digestion than milk. In fact, it seldom disagrees. Cheese is not usually digestible by the sick, but it is pure nourishment for repairing waste; and I have seen sick, and not a few either, whose craving for cheese shewed how much it was needed by them.＊

But, if fresh milk is so valuable a food for the sick, the least change or sourness in it, makes it of all articles, perhaps, the most injurious; diarrhœa is a common result of fresh milk allowed to become at all sour. The nurse therefore ought to exercise her utmost care in this. In large institutions for the sick, even the poorest, the utmost care is exercised. Wenham Lake ice is used for this express purpose every summer, while the private patient, perhaps, never tastes a drop of milk that is not sour, all through the hot weather, so little does the private nurse understand the necessity of such care. Yet, if you consider that the only drop of real nourishment in your patient's tea is the drop of milk, and how much almost all English patients depend

Intelligent cravings of particular sick for particular articles of diet.

＊ In the diseases produced by bad food, such as scorbutic dysentery and diarrhœa, the patient's stomach often craves for and digests things, some of which certainly would be laid down in no dietary that ever was invented for sick, and especially not for such sick. These are fruit, pickles, jams, gingerbread, fat of ham or of bacon, suet, cheese, butter, milk. These cases I have seen not by ones, nor by tens, but by hundreds. And the patient's stomach was right and the book was wrong. The articles craved for, in these cases, might have been principall arranged under the two heads of fat and vegetable acids.
There is often a marked difference between men and women in this matter of sick feeding. Women's digestion is generally slower.

upon their tea, you will see the great importance of not depriving your patient of this drop of milk. Buttermilk, a totally different thing, is often very useful, especially in fevers.

In laying down rules of diet, by the amounts of " solid nutri- Sweet things ment " in different kinds of food, it is constantly lost sight of what the patient requires to repair his waste, what he can take and what he can't. You cannot diet a patient from a book, you cannot make up the human body as you would make up a prescription,—so many parts " carboniferous," so many parts " nitrogenous " will consti- tute a perfect diet for the patient. The nurse's observation here will materially assist the doctor—the patient's " fancies " will materially assist the nurse. For instance, sugar is one of the most nutritive of all articles, being pure carbon, and is particularly recom- mended in some books. But the vast majority of all patients in England, young and old, male and female, rich and poor, hospital and private, dislike sweet things,—and while I have never known a person take to sweets when he was ill who disliked them when he was well, I have known many fond of them when in health, who in sickness would leave off anything sweet, even to sugar in tea,—sweet puddings, sweet drinks, are their aversion; the furred tongue almost always likes what is sharp or pungent. Scorbutic patients are an exception, they often crave for sweetmeats and jams.

Jelly is another article of diet in great favour with nurses and friends of the sick; even if it could be eaten solid, it would not nourish, but it is simply the height of folly to take $\frac{1}{8}$ oz. of gelatine and make it into a certain bulk by dissolving it in water and then to give it to the sick, as if the mere bulk represented nourishment. It is now known that jelly does not nourish, that it has a tendency to produce diarrhœa,—and to trust to it to repair the waste of a diseased constitution is simply to starve the sick under the guise of feeding them. If 100 spoonfuls of jelly were given in the course of the day, you would have given one spoonful of gelatine, which spoonful has no nutritive power whatever.

And, nevertheless, gelatine contains a large quantity of nitrogen, which is one of the most powerful elements in nutrition; on the other hand, beef tea may be chosen as an illustration of great nutrient power in sickness, co-existing with a very small amount of solid nitrogenous matter.

Dr. Christison says that " every one will be struck with the readi- Beef tea. ness with which " certain classes of " patients will often take diluted meat juice or beef tea repeatedly, when they refuse all other kinds of food." This is particularly remarkable in " cases of gastric fever, in which," he says, " little or nothing else besides beef tea or diluted meat juice " has been taken for weeks or even months, " and yet a pint of beef tea contains scarcely $\frac{1}{4}$ oz. of anything but water,"—the result is so striking that he asks what is its mode of action ? " Not simply nutrient—$\frac{1}{4}$ oz. of the most nutritive material cannot nearly replace the daily wear and tear of the tissues in any circumstances. Possibly," he says, " it belongs to a new denomination of remedies."

It has been observed that a small quantity of beef tea added to other articles of nutrition augments their power out of all proportion to the additional amount of solid matter.

The reason why jelly should be innutritious and beef tea nutritious to the sick, is a secret yet undiscovered, but it clearly shows that careful observation of the sick is the only clue to the best dietary.

Observation, not chemistry, must decide sick diet. Chemistry has as yet afforded little insight into the dieting of sick. All that chemistry can tell us is the amount of "carboniferous" or "nitrogenous" elements discoverable in different dietetic articles. It has given us lists of dietetic substances, arranged in the order of their richness in one or other of these principles; but that is all. In the great majority of cases, the stomach of the patient is guided by other principles of selection than merely the amount of carbon or nitrogen in the diet. No doubt, in this as in other things, nature has very definite rules for her guidance, but these rules can only be ascertained by the most careful observation at the bed-side. She there teaches us that living chemistry, the chemistry of reparation, is something different from the chemistry of the laboratory. Organic chemistry is useful, as all knowledge is, when we come face to face with nature; but it by no means follows that we should learn in the laboratory any one of the reparative processes going on in disease.

Again, the nutritive power of milk and of the preparations from milk, is very much undervalued; there is nearly as much nourishment in half a pint of milk as there is in a quarter of a lb. of meat. But this is not the whole question or nearly the whole. The main question is what the patient's stomach can assimilate or derive nourishment from, and of this the patient's stomach is the sole judge. Chemistry cannot tell this. The patient's stomach must be its own chemist. The diet which will keep the healthy man healthy, will kill the sick one. The same beef which is the most nutritive of all meat and which nourishes the healthy man, is the least nourishing of all food to the sick man, whose half-dead stomach can *assimilate* no part of it, that is, make no food out of it. On a diet of beef tea healthy men on the other hand speedily lose their strength.

Home-made bread. I have known patients live for many months without touching bread, because they could not eat baker's bread. These were mostly country patients, but not all. Home-made bread or brown bread is a most important article of diet for many patients. The use of aperients may be entirely superseded by it. Oat cake is another.

Sound observation has scarcely yet been brought to bear on sick diet. To watch for the opinions, then, which the patient's stomach gives, rather than to read "analyses of foods," is the business of all those who have to settle what the patient is to eat—perhaps the most important thing to be provided for him after the air he is to breathe. Now the medical man who sees the patient only once a day or even only once or twice a week, cannot possibly tell this without the assistance of the patient himself, or of those who are in constant observation on the patient. The utmost the medical man can tell is whether the patient is weaker or stronger at this visit than he was at the last visit. I should therefore say that incomparably the most important office of the nurse, after she has taken care of the patient's

[Original page no. 42]

air, is to take care to observe the effect of his food, and report it to the medical attendant.

It is quite incalculable the good that would certainly come from such *sound* and close observation in this almost neglected branch of nursing, or the help it would give to the medical man.

A great deal too much against tea* is said by wise people, and a Tea and coffee. great deal too much of tea is given to the sick by foolish people. When you see the natural and almost universal craving in English sick for their "tea," you cannot but feel that nature knows what she is about. But a little tea or coffee restores them quite as much as a great deal, and a great deal of tea and especially of coffee impairs the little power of digestion they have. Yet a nurse because she sees how one or two cups of tea or coffee restores her patient, thinks that three or four cups will do twice as much. This is not the case at all; it is however certain that there is nothing yet discovered which is a substitute to the English patient for his cup of tea; he can take it when he can take nothing else, and he often can't take anything else if he has it not. I should be very glad if any of the abusers of tea would point out what to give to an English patient after a sleepless night, instead of tea. If you give it at 5 or 6 o'clock in the morning, he may even sometimes fall asleep after it, and get perhaps his only two or three hours' sleep during the twenty-four. At the same time you never should give tea or coffee to the sick, as a rule, after 5 o'clock in the afternoon. Sleeplessness in the early night is from excitement generally and is increased by tea or coffee; sleeplessness which continues to the early morning is from exhaustion often, and is relieved by tea. The only English patients I have ever known refuse tea, have been typhus cases, and the first sign of their getting better was their craving again for tea. In general, the dry and dirty tongue always prefers tea to coffee, and will quite decline milk, unless with tea. Coffee is a better restorative than tea, but a

---

* It is made a frequent recommendation to persons about to incur great exhaustion, either from the nature of the service or from their being not in a state fit for it, to eat a piece of bread before they go. I wish the recommenders would themselves try the experiment of substituting a piece of bread for a cup of tea or coffee or beef tea as a refresher. They would find it a very poor comfort. When soldiers have to set out fasting on fatiguing duty, when nurses have to go fasting in to their patients, it is a hot restorative they want, and ought to have, before they go, not a cold bit of bread. And dreadful have been the consequences of neglecting this. If they can take a bit of bread *with* the hot cup of tea, so much the better, but not *instead* of it. The fact that there is more nourishment in bread than in almost anything else has probably induced the mistake. That it is a fatal mistake there is no doubt. It seems, though very little is known on the subject, that what "assimilates" itself directly and with the least trouble of digestion with the human body is the best for the above circumstances. Bread requires two or three processes of assimilation, before it becomes like the human body.

The almost universal testimony of English men and women who have undergone great fatigue, such as riding long journeys without stopping, or sitting up for several nights in succession, is that they could do it best upon an occasional cup of tea—and nothing else.

Let experience, not theory, decide upon this as upon all other things.

greater impairer of the digestion. Let the patient's taste decide. You will say that, in cases of great thirst, the patient's craving decides that it will drink *a great deal* of tea, and that you cannot help it. But in these cases be sure that the patient requires diluents for quite other purposes than quenching the thirst; he wants a great deal of some drink, not only of tea, and the doctor will order what he is to have, barley water or lemonade, or soda water and milk, as the case may be.

Lehmann, quoted by Dr. Christison, says that, among the well and active "the infusion of 1 oz. of roasted coffee daily will diminish the waste" going on in the body "by one-fourth," and Dr. Christison adds that tea has the same property. Now this is actual experiment. Lehmann weighs the man and finds the fact from his weight. It is not deduced from any "analysis" of food. All experience among the sick shows the same thing.*

Cocoa.

Cocoa is often recommended to the sick in lieu of tea or coffee. But independently of the fact that English sick very generally dislike cocoa, it has quite a different effect from tea or coffee. It is an oily starchy nut having no restorative power at all, but simply increasing fat. It is pure mockery of the sick, therefore, to call it a substitute for tea. For any renovating stimulus it has, you might just as well offer them chestnuts instead of tea.

Bulk.

An almost universal error among nurses is in the bulk of the food and especially the drinks they offer to their patients Suppose a patient ordered 4 oz. brandy during the day, how is he to take this if you make it into four pints with diluting it? The same with tea and beef tea, with arrowroot, milk, &c. You have not increased the nourishment, you have not increased the renovating power of these articles, by increasing their bulk,—you have very likely diminished both by giving the patient's digestion more to do, and most likely of all, the patient will leave half of what he has been ordered to take, because he cannot swallow the bulk with which you have been pleased to invest it. It requires very nice observation and care (and meets with hardly any) to determine what will not be too thick or strong for the patient to take, while giving him no more than the bulk which he is able to swallow.

* In making coffee, it is absolutely necessary to buy it in the berry and grind it at home. Otherwise you may reckon upon its containing a certain amount of chicory, *at least*. This is not a question of the taste or of the wholesomeness of chicory. It is that chicory has nothing at all of the properties for which you give coffee. And therefore you may as well not give it.

Again, all laundresses, mistresses of dairy-farms, head nurses (I speak of the good old sort only—women who unite a good deal of hard manual labour with the head-work necessary for arranging the day's business, so that none of it shall tread upon the heels of something else) set great value, I have observed, upon having a high-priced tea. This is called extravagant. But these women are "extravagant" in nothing else. And they are right in this. Real tea-leaf tea alone contains the restorative they want; which is not to be found in sloe-leaf tea.

The mistresses of houses, who cannot even go over their own house once a-day, are incapable of judging for these women. For they are incapable themselves, to all appearance, of the spirit of arrangement (no small task) necessary for managing a large ward or dairy.

VIII. BED AND BEDDING.

A few words upon bedsteads and bedding; and principally as **Feverishness** regards patients who are entirely, or almost entirely, confined to bed. **a symptom of** Feverishness is generally supposed to be a symptom of fever— **bedding.** in nine cases out of ten it is a symptom of bedding.* The patient has had re-introduced into the body the emanations from himself which day after day and week after week saturate his unaired bedding. How can it be otherwise? Look at the ordinary bed in which a patient lies.

If I were looking out for an example in order to show what *not* **Uncleanliness** to do, I should take the specimen of an ordinary bed in a private **of ordinary** house: a wooden bedstead, two or even three mattresses piled up to **bedding.** above the height of a table; a vallance attached to the frame— nothing but a miracle could ever thoroughly dry or air such a bed and bedding. The patient must inevitably alternate between cold damp after his bed is made, and warm damp before, both saturated with organic matter,† and this from the time the mattresses are put under him till the time they are picked to pieces, if this is ever done.

If you consider that an adult in health exhales by the lungs and **Air your dirty** skin in the twenty-four hours three pints at least of moisture, loaded **sheets, not** with organic matter ready to enter into putrefaction; that in sickness **only your** the quantity is often greatly increased, the quality is always more **clean ones.** noxious—just ask yourself next where does all this moisture go to? Chiefly into the bedding, because it cannot go anywhere else. And it stays there; because, except perhaps a weekly change of sheets, scarcely any other airing is attempted. A nurse will be careful to fidgetiness about airing the clean sheets from clean damp, but airing the dirty sheets from noxious damp will never even occur to her. Besides this, the most dangerous effluvia we know of are from the excreta of the sick—these are placed, at least temporarily, where they must throw their effluvia into the under side of the bed, and the space under the bed is never aired; it cannot be, with our arrangements. Must not such a bed be always saturated, and be always the means of re-introducing into the system of the unfortunate patient who lies in it, that excrementitious matter to eliminate which from the body nature had expressly appointed the disease?

My heart always sinks within me when I hear the good housewife, of every class, say, "I assure you the bed has been well slept

* I once told a "very good nurse" that the way in which her patient's room **Nurses often** was kept was quite enough to account for his sleeplessness; and she answered **do not think** quite good-humouredly she was not at all surprised at it—as if the state of the **the sick-room** room were, like the state of the weather, entirely out of her power. Now in what **any business of** sense was this woman to be called a "nurse"? **theirs, but**

† For the same reason if, after washing a patient, you must put the same **only the sick.** night-dress on him again, always give it a preliminary warm at the fire. The night-gown he has worn must be, to a certain extent, damp. It has now got cold from having been off him for a few minutes. The fire will dry and at the same time air it. This is much more important than with clean things.

[Original page no. 45]

in," and I can only hope it is not true. What? is the bed already saturated with somebody else's damp before my patient comes to exhale into it his own damp? Has it not had a single chance to be aired? No, not one. "It has been slept in every night."

Iron spring bedstead the best.

The only way of really nursing a real patient is to have an *iron* bedstead, with rheocline springs, which are permeable by the air up to the very mattress (no vallance, of course), the mattress to be a thin hair one; the bed to be not above 3½ feet wide. If the patient

Comfort and cleanliness of *two* beds.

be entirely confined to his bed; there should be *two* such bedsteads; each bed to be "made" with mattress, sheets, blankets, &c., complete —the patient to pass twelve hours in each bed; on no account to carry his sheets with him. The whole of the bedding to be hung up to air for each intermediate twelve hours. Of course there are many cases where this cannot be done at all—many more where only an approach to it can be made. I am indicating the ideal of nursing, and what I have actually had done. But about the kind of bedstead there can be no doubt, whether there be one or two provided.

Bed not to be too wide.

There is a prejudice in favour of a wide bed—I believe it to be a prejudice. All the refreshment of moving a patient from one side to the other of his bed is far more effectually secured by putting him into a fresh bed; and a patient who is really very ill does not stray far in bed. But it is said there is no room to put a tray down on a narrow bed. No good nurse will ever put a tray on a bed at all. If the patient can turn on his side, he will eat more comfortably from a bed-side table; and on no account whatever should a bed ever be higher than a sofa. Otherwise the patient feels himself "out of humanity's reach"; he can get at nothing for himself: he can move nothing for himself. If the patient cannot turn, a table over the bed is a better thing. I need hardly say that a patient's bed should never have its side against the wall. The nurse must be able to get easily to both sides the bed, and to reach easily every part of the patient without stretching—a thing impossible if the bed be either too wide or too high.

Bed not to be too high.

When I see a patient in a room nine or ten feet high upon a bed between four and five feet high, with his head, when he is sitting up in bed, actually within two or three feet of the ceiling, I ask myself, is this expressly planned to produce that peculiarly distressing feeling common to the sick, viz., as if the walls and ceiling were closing in upon them, and they becoming sandwiches between floor and ceiling, which imagination is not, indeed, here so far from the truth? If, over and above this, the window stops short of the ceiling, then the patient's head may literally be raised above the stratum of fresh air, even when the window is open. Can human perversity any farther go, in unmaking the process of restoration which God has made? The fact is, that the heads of sleepers or of sick should never be higher than the throat of the chimney, which ensures their being in the current of best air. And we will not suppose it possible that you have closed your chimney with a chimney-board.

If a bed is higher than a sofa, the difference of the fatigue of getting in and out of bed will just make the difference, very often, to the patient (who can get in and out of bed at all) of being able to take a few minutes' exercise, either in the open air or in another room. It is so very odd that people never think of this, or of how many more times a patient who is in bed for the twenty-four hours is obliged to get in and out of bed than they are, who only, it is to be hoped, get into bed once and out of bed once during the twenty-four hours.

A patient's bed should always be in the lightest spot in the room; and he should be able to see out of window.

Nor in a dark place.

I need scarcely say that the old four-post bed with curtains is utterly inadmissible, whether for sick or well. Hospital bedsteads are in many respects very much less objectionable than private ones.

Nor a four poster with curtains.

There is reason to believe that not a few of the apparently unaccountable cases of scrofula among children proceed from the habit of sleeping with the head under the bed clothes, and so inhaling air already breathed, which is farther contaminated by exhalations from the skin. Patients are sometimes given to a similar habit, and it often happens that the bed clothes are so disposed that the patient must necessarily breathe air more or less contaminated by exhalations from his skin. A good nurse will be careful to attend to this. It is an important part, so to speak, of ventilation.

Scrofula often a result of disposition of bedclothes.

It may be worth while to remark, that where there is any danger of bed-sores a blanket should never be placed *under* the patient. It retains damp and acts like a poultice.

Bed sores.

Never use anything but light Witney blankets as bed covering for the sick. The heavy cotton impervious counterpane is bad, for the very reason that it keeps in the emanations from the sick person, while the blanket allows them to pass through. Weak patients are invariably distressed by a great weight of bed-clothes, which often prevents their getting any sound sleep whatever.

Heavy and impervious bedclothes.

NOTE.—One word about pillows. Every weak patient, be his illness what it may, suffers more or less from difficulty in breathing. To take the weight of the body off the poor chest, which is hardly up to its work as it is, ought therefore to be the object of the nurse in arranging his pillows. Now what does she do and what are the consequences? She piles the pillows one a-top of the other like a wall of bricks. The head is thrown upon the chest. And the shoulders are pushed forward, so as not to allow the lungs room to expand. The pillows, in fact, lean upon the patient, not the patient upon the pillows. It is impossible to give a rule for this, because it must vary with the figure of the patient. And tall patients suffer much more than short ones, because of the *drag* of the long limbs upon the waist. But the object is to support, with the pillows, the back *below* the breathing apparatus, to allow the shoulders room to fall back, and to support the head, without throwing it forward. The suffering of dying patients is immensely increased by neglect of these points. And many an invalid, too weak to drag about his pillows himself, slips his book or anything at hand behind the lower part of his back to support it.

IX. LIGHT.

It is the unqualified result of all my experience with the sick, that second only to their need of fresh air is their need of light;

Light essential to both health and recovery.

[Original page no. 47]

that, after a close room, what hurts them most is a dark room. And that it is not only light but direct sun-light they want. I had rather have the power of carrying my patient about after the sun, according to the aspect of the rooms, if circumstances permit, than let him linger in a room when the sun is off. People think the effect is upon the spirits only. This is by no means the case. The sun is not only a painter but a sculptor. You admit that he does the photograph. Without going into any scientific exposition we must admit that light has quite as real and tangible effects upon the human body. But this is not all. Who has not observed the purifying effect of light, and especially of direct sunlight, upon the air of a room? Here is an observation within everybody's experience. Go into a room where the shutters are always shut, (in a sick room or a bedroom there should never be shutters shut), and though the room be uninhabited, though the air has never been polluted by the breathing of human beings, you will observe a close, musty smell of corrupt air, of air i. e. unpurified by the effect of the sun's rays. The mustiness of dark rooms and corners, indeed, is proverbial. The cheerfulness of a room, the usefulness of light in treating disease is all-important.

Aspect, view, and sunlight matters of first importance to the sick.

A very high authority in hospital construction has said that people do not enough consider the difference between wards and dormitories in planning their buildings. But I go farther, and say, that healthy people never remember the difference between *bed*-rooms and *sick*-rooms, in making arrangements for the sick. To a sleeper in health it does not signify what the view is from his bed. He ought never to be in it excepting when asleep, and at night. Aspect does not very much signify either (provided the sun reach his bed-room some time in every day, to purify the air), because he ought never to be in his bed-room except during the hours when there is no sun. But the case is exactly reversed with the sick, even should they be as many hours out of their beds as you are in yours, which probably they are not. Therefore, that they should be able, without raising themselves or turning in bed, to see out of window from their beds, to see sky and sun-light at least, if you can show them nothing else, I assert to be, if not of the very first importance for recovery, at least something very near it. And you should therefore look to the position of the beds of your sick one of the very first things. If they can see out of two windows instead of one, so much the better. Again, the morning sun and the mid-day sun—the hours when they are quite certain not to be up, are of more importance to them, if a choice must be made, than the afternoon sun. Perhaps you can take them out of bed in the afternoon and set them by the window, where they can see the sun. But the best rule is, if possible, to give them direct sun-light from the moment he rises till the moment he sets.

Another great difference between the *bed*-room and the *sick*-room is, that the *sleeper* has a very large balance of fresh air to begin with, when he begins the night, if his room has been open all day as it ought to be; the *sick* man has not, because all day he has been breathing the air in the same room, and dirtying it by the emanations from himself. Far more care is therefore necessary to keep up a constant change of air in the sick room.

It is hardly necessary to add that there are acute cases, (particularly a few ophthalmic cases, and diseases where the eye is morbidly sensitive), where a subdued light is necessary. But a dark north room is inadmissible even for these. You can always moderate the light by blinds and curtains.

Heavy, thick, dark window or bed curtains should, however, hardly ever be used for any kind of sick in this country. A light white curtain at the head of the bed is, in general, all that is necessary, and a green blind to the window, to be drawn down only when necessary.

One of the greatest observers of human things (not physiological), says, in another language, "Where there is sun there is thought." All physiology goes to confirm this. Where is the shady side of deep valleys, there is cretinism. Where are cellars and the unsunned sides of narrow streets, there is the degeneracy and weakliness of the human race—mind and body equally degenerating. Put the pale withering plant and human being into the sun, and, if not too far gone, each will recover health and spirit. *Without sunlight, we degenerate body and mind.*

It is a curious thing to observe how almost all patients lie with their faces turned to the light, exactly as plants always make their way towards the light; a patient will even complain that it gives him pain "lying on that side." "Then why *do* you lie on that side?" He does not know,—but we do. It is because it is the side towards the window. A fashionable physician has recently published in a government report that he always turns his patients' faces from the light. Yes, but nature is stronger than fashionable physicians, and depend upon it she turns the faces back and *towards* such light as she can get. Walk through the wards of a hospital, remember the bed sides of private patients you have seen, and count how many sick you ever saw lying with their faces towards the wall. *Almost all patients lie with their faces to the light.*

X. CLEANLINESS OF ROOMS AND WALLS.

It cannot be necessary to tell a nurse that she should be clean, or that she should keep her patient clean,—seeing that the greater part of nursing consists in preserving cleanliness. No ventilation can freshen a room or ward where the most scrupulous cleanliness is not observed. Unless the wind be blowing through the windows at the rate of twenty miles an hour, dusty carpets, dirty wainscots, musty curtains and furniture, will infallibly produce a close smell. I have lived in a large and expensively furnished London house, where the only constant inmate in two very lofty rooms, with opposite windows, was myself, and yet, owing to the abovementioned dirty circumstances, no opening of windows could ever keep those *Cleanliness of carpets and furniture.*

rooms free from closeness.; but the carpet and curtains having been turned out of the rooms altogether, they became instantly as fresh as could be wished. It is pure nonsense to say that in London a room cannot be kept clean. Many of our hospitals show the exact reverse.

Dust never removed now. But no particle of dust is ever or can ever be removed or really got rid of by the present system of dusting. Dusting in these days means nothing but flapping the dust from one part of a room on to another with doors and windows closed. What you do it for I cannot think. You had much better leave the dust alone, if you are not going to take it away altogether. For from the time a room begins to be a room up to the time when it ceases to be one, no one atom of dust ever actually leaves its precincts. Tidying a room means nothing now but removing a thing from one place, which it has kept clean for itself, on to another and a dirtier one.* Flapping by way of cleaning is only admissible in the case of pictures, or anything made of paper. The only way I know to *remove* dust, the plague of all lovers of fresh air, is to wipe everything with a damp cloth. And all furniture ought to be so made as that it may be wiped with a damp cloth without injury to itself, and so polished as that it may be damped without injury to others. To dust, as it is now practised, truly means to distribute dust more equally over a room.

Floors. As to floors, the only really clean floor I know is the Berlin *lackered* floor, which is wet rubbed and dry rubbed every morning to remove the dust. The French *parquet* is always more or less dusty, although infinitely superior in point of cleanliness and healthiness to our absorbent floor.

For a sick room, a carpet is perhaps the worst expedient which could by any possibility have been invented. If you must have a carpet, the only safety is to take it up two or three times a year, instead of once. A dirty carpet literally infects the room. And if you consider the enormous quantity of organic matter from the feet of people coming in, which must saturate it, this is by no means surprising.

Papered, plastered, oil-painted walls. As for walls, the worst is the papered wall; the next worst is plaster. But the plaster can be redeemed by frequent lime-washing; the paper requires frequent renewing. A glazed paper gets rid of a

How a room is dusted. * If you like to clean your furniture by laying out your clean clothes upon your dirty chairs or sofa, this is one way certainly of doing it. Having witnessed the morning process called "tidying the room," for many years, and with ever-increasing astonishment, I can describe what it is. From the chairs, tables, or sofa, upon which the "things" have lain during the night, and which are therefore comparatively clean from dust or blacks, the poor "*things*" having "caught" it, they are removed to other chairs, tables, sofas, upon which you could write your name with your finger in the dust or blacks. The *other* side of the "things" is therefore now evenly dirtied or dusted. The housemaid then flaps every thing, or some things, not out of her reach, with a thing called a duster— the dust flies up, then re-settles more equally than it lay before the operation. The room has now been "put to rights."

good deal of the danger. But the ordinary bed-room paper is all that it ought *not* to be.*

The close connection between ventilation and cleanliness is shown in this. An ordinary light paper will last clean much longer if there is an Arnott's ventilator in the chimney than it otherwise would.

The best wall now extant is oil paint. From this you can wash the animal exuviæ.†

These are what make a room musty.

The best wall for a sick-room or ward that could be made is pure white non-absorbent cement or glass, or glazed tiles, if they were made sightly enough. Best kind of wall for a sick-room.

Air can be soiled just like water. If you blow into water you will soil it with the animal matter from your breath. So it is with air. Air is always soiled in a room where walls and carpets are saturated with animal exhalations.

Want of cleanliness, then, in rooms and wards, which you have to guard against, may arise in three ways.

1. Dirty air coming in from without, soiled by sewer emanations, the evaporation from dirty streets, smoke, bits of unburnt fuel, bits of straw, bits of horse dung. Dirty air from without.

If people would but cover the outside walls of their houses with plain or encaustic tiles, what an incalculable improvement would there be in light, cleanliness, dryness, warmth, and consequently economy. The play of a fire-engine would then effectually wash the outside of a house. This kind of *walling* would stand next to paving in improving the health of towns. Best kind of wall for a house.

2. Dirty air coming from within, from dust, which you often displace, but never remove. And this recalls what ought to be a *sine qua non.* Have as few ledges in your room or ward as possible. And under no pretence have any ledge whatever out of sight. Dust accumulates there, and will never be wiped off. This is a certain way to soil the air. Besides this, the animal exhalations from your inmates saturate your furniture. And if you never clean your furniture properly, how can your rooms or wards be anything but musty? Ventilate as you please, the rooms will never be sweet. Besides this, there is a constant *degradation,* as it is called, taking place from everything except polished or glazed articles—*E. g.*, in colouring certain green papers arsenic is used. Now in the very dust even, which is lying about in rooms hung with this kind of green paper, arsenic has been distinctly detected. You see your dust is anything but harmless; yet you will let such dust lie about your ledges for months, your rooms for ever. Dirty air from within.

Atmosphere in painted and papered rooms quite distinguishable.

* I am sure that a person who has accustomed her senses to compare atmospheres proper and improper, for the sick and for children, could tell, blindfold, the difference of the air in old painted and in old papered rooms, *cæteris paribus.* The latter will always be musty, even with all the windows open.

† If you like to wipe your dirty door, or some portion of your dirty wall, by hanging up your clean gown or shawl against it on a peg, this is one way certainly, and the most usual way, and generally the only way of cleaning either door or wall in a bed-room! How to keep your wall clean at the expence of your clothes.

Again, the fire fills the room with coal-dust.

Dirty air from the carpet.

3. Dirty air coming from the carpet. Above all, take care of the carpets, that the animal dirt left there by the feet of visitors does not stay there. Floors, unless the grain is filled up and polished, are just as bad. The smell from the floor of a school-room or ward, when any moisture brings out the organic matter by which it is saturated, might alone be enough to warn us of the mischief that is going on.

Remedies.

The outer air, then, can only be kept clean by sanitary improvements, and by consuming smoke. The expense in soap, which this single improvement would save, is quite incalculable.

The inside air can only be kept clean by excessive care in the ways mentioned above—to rid the walls, carpets, furniture, ledges, &c., of the organic matter and dust—dust consisting greatly of this organic matter—with which they become saturated, and which is what really makes the room musty.

Without cleanliness, you cannot have all the effect of ventilation; without ventilation, you can have no thorough cleanliness.

Very few people, be they of what class they may, have any idea of the exquisite cleanliness required in the sick-room. For much of what I have said applies less to the hospital than to the private sick-room. The smoky chimney, the dusty furniture, the utensils emptied but once a day, often keep the air of the sick constantly dirty in the best private houses.

The well have a curious habit of forgetting that what is to them but a trifling inconvenience, to be patiently " put up " with, is to the sick a source of suffering, delaying recovery, if not actually hastening death. The well are scarcely ever more than eight hours, at most, in the same room. Some change they can always make, if only for a few minutes. Even during the supposed eight hours, they can change their posture or their position in the room. But the sick man, who never leaves his bed, who cannot change by any movement of his own his air, or his light, or his warmth; who cannot obtain quiet, or get out of the smoke, or the smell, or the dust; he is really poisoned or depressed by what is to you the merest trifle.

" What can't be cured must be endured," is the very worst and most dangerous maxim for a nurse which ever was made. Patience and resignation in her are but other words for carelessness or indifference—contemptible, if in regard to herself; culpable, if in regard to her sick.

XI. PERSONAL CLEANLINESS.

Poisoning by the skin.

In almost all diseases, the function of the skin is, more or less, disordered; and in many most important diseases nature relieves herself almost entirely by the skin. This is particularly the case with children. But the excretion, which comes from the skin, is left there, unless removed by washing or by the clothes. Every nurse.

should keep this fact constantly in mind,—for, if she allow her sick to remain unwashed, or their clothing to remain on them after being saturated with perspiration or other excretion, she is interfering injuriously with the natural processes of health just as effectually as if she were to give the patient a dose of slow poison by the mouth. Poisoning by the skin is no less certain than poisoning by the mouth —only it is slower in its operation.

The amount of relief and comfort experienced by sick after the skin has been carefully washed and dried, is one of the commonest observations made at a sick bed. But it must not be forgotten that the comfort and relief so obtained are not all. They are, in fact, nothing more than a sign that the vital powers have been relieved by removing something that was oppressing them. The nurse, therefore, must never put off attending to the personal cleanliness of her patient under the plea that all that is to be gained is a little relief, which can be quite as well given later. *[Ventilation and skin-cleanliness equally essential.]*

In all well-regulated hospitals this ought to be, and generally is, attended to. But it is very generally neglected with private sick.

Just as it is necessary to renew the air round a sick person frequently, to carry off morbid effluvia from the lungs and skin, by maintaining free ventilation, so is it necessary to keep the pores of the skin free from all obstructing excretions. The object, both of ventilation and of skin-cleanliness, is pretty much the same,—to wit, removing noxious matter from the system as rapidly as possible.

Care should be taken in all these operations of sponging, washing, and cleansing the skin, not to expose too great a surface at once, so as to check the perspiration, which would renew the evil in another form.

The various ways of washing the sick need not here be specified, —the less so as the doctors ought to say which is to be used.

In several forms of diarrhœa, dysentery, &c., where the skin is hard and harsh, the relief afforded by washing with a great deal of soft soap is incalculable. In other cases, sponging with tepid soap and water, then with tepid water and drying with a hot towel will be ordered.

Every nurse ought to be careful to wash her hands very frequently during the day. If her face too, so much the better.

One word as to cleanliness merely as cleanliness.

Compare the dirtiness of the water in which you have washed when it is cold without soap, cold with soap, hot with soap. You will find the first has hardly removed any dirt at all, the second a little more, the third a great deal more. But hold your hand over a cup of hot water for a minute or two, and then, by merely rubbing with the finger, you will bring off flakes of dirt or dirty skin. After a vapour bath you may peel your whole self clean in this way. What I mean is, that by simply washing or sponging with water you do not really clean your skin. Take a rough towel, dip one corner in very hot water,—if a little spirit be added to it it will be more effectual,— and then rub as if you were rubbing the towel into your skin with your fingers. The black flakes which will come off will convince *[Steaming and rubbing the skin.]*

you that you were not clean before, however much soap and water you have used. These flakes are what require removing. And you can really keep yourself cleaner with a tumbler of hot water and a rough towel and rubbing, than with a whole apparatus of bath and soap and sponge, without rubbing. It is quite nonsense to say that anybody need be dirty. Patients have been kept as clean by these means on a long voyage, when a basin full of water could not be afforded, and when they could not be moved out of their berths, as if all the appurtenances of home had been at hand.

Washing, however, with a large quantity of water has quite other effects than those of mere cleanliness. The skin absorbs the water and becomes softer and more perspirable. To wash with soap and soft water is, therefore, desirable from other points of view than that of cleanliness.

XII. CHATTERING HOPES AND ADVICES.

Advising the sick.

The sick man to his advisers.

"My advisers ! Their name is legion.   *   *   *
Somehow or other, it seems a provision of the universal destinies, that every man, woman, and child should consider him, her, or itself privileged especially to advise me. Why ? That is precisely what I want to know." And this is what I have to say to them. I have been advised to go to every place extant in and out of England—to take every kind of exercise by every kind of cart, carriage—yes, and even swing (!) and dumb-bell (!) in existence; to imbibe every different kind of stimulus that ever has been invented. And this when those *best* fitted to know, viz., medical men, after long and close attendance, had declared any journey out of the question, had prohibited any kind of motion whatever, had closely laid down the diet and drink. What would my advisers say, were they the medical attendants, and I the patient left their advice, and took the casual adviser's ? But the singularity in Legion's mind is this : it never occurs to him that everybody else is doing the same thing, and that I the patient *must* perforce say, in sheer self-defence, like Rosalind, "I could not do with all."

Chattering hopes the bane of the sick.

"Chattering Hopes" may seem an odd heading. But I really believe there is scarcely a greater worry which invalids have to endure than the incurable hopes of their friends. There is no one practice against which I can speak more strongly from actual personal experience, wide and long, of its effects during sickness observed both upon others and upon myself. I would appeal most seriously to all friends, visitors, and attendants of the sick to leave off this practice of attempting to "cheer" the sick by making light of their danger and by exaggerating their probabilities of recovery.

Far more now than formerly does the medical attendant tell the truth to the sick who are really desirous to hear it about their own state.

How intense is the folly, then, to say the least of it, of the friend, be he even a medical man, who thinks that his opinion, given after a cursory observation, will weigh with the patient, against the opinion of the medical attendant, given, perhaps, after years of observation, after using every help to diagnosis afforded by the stethoscope, the examination of pulse, tongue, &c.; and certainly after much more observation than the friend can possibly have had.

Supposing the patient to be possessed of common sense,—how can the "favourable" opinion, if it is to be called an opinion at all, of the casual visitor "cheer" him,—when different from that of the experienced attendant? Unquestionably the latter may, and often does, turn out to be wrong. But which is most likely to be wrong?

The fact is, that the patient* is not "cheered" at all by these well-meaning, most tiresome friends. On the contrary, he is depressed and wearied. If, on the one hand, he exerts himself to tell each successive member of this too numerous conspiracy, whose name is legion, why he does not think as they do,—in what respect he is worse,—what symptoms exist that they know nothing of,—he is fatigued instead of "cheered," and his attention is fixed upon himself. In general, patients who are really ill, do not want to talk about themselves. Hypochondriacs do, but again I say we are not on the subject of hypochondriacs. `Patient does not want to talk of himself.`

If, on the other hand, and which is much more frequently the case, the patient says nothing, but the Shakespearian "Oh!" "Ah!" "Go to!" and "In good sooth!" in order to escape from the conversation about himself the sooner, he is depressed by want of sympathy. He feels isolated in the midst of friends. He feels what a convenience it would be, if there were any single person to whom he could speak simply and openly, without pulling the string upon himself of this `Absurd consolations put forth for the benefit of the sick.`

* There are, of course cases, as in first confinements, when an assurance from the doctor or experienced nurse to the frightened suffering woman that there is nothing unusual in her case, that she has nothing to fear but a few hours' pain, may cheer her most effectually. This is advice of quite another order. It is the advice of experience to utter inexperience. But the advice we have been referring to is the advice of inexperience to bitter experience; and, in general, amounts to nothing more than this, that *you* think *I* shall recover from consumption, because somebody knows somebody somewhere who has recovered from fever. `Absurd statistical comparisons made in common conversation by the most sensible people for the benefit of the sick.`

I have heard a doctor condemned whose patient did not, alas! recover, because another doctor's patient of a *different* sex, of a *different* age, recovered from a *different* disease, in a *different* place. Yes, this is really true. If people who make these comparisons did but know (only they do not care to know), the care and preciseness with which such comparisons require to be made, (and are made), in order to be of any value whatever, they would spare their tongues. In comparing the deaths of one hospital with those of another, any statistics are justly considered absolutely valueless which do not give the ages, the sexes, and the diseases of all the cases. It does not seem necessary to mention this. It does not seem necessary to say that there can be no comparison between old men with dropsies and young women with consumptions. Yet the cleverest men and the cleverest women are often heard making such comparisons, ignoring entirely sex, age, disease, place—in fact, *all* the conditions essential to the question. It is the merest *gossip*.

shower-bath of silly hopes and encouragements; to whom he could express his wishes and directions without that person persisting in saying "I hope that it will please God yet to give you twenty years," or, "You have a long life of activity before you." How often we see at the end of biographies or of cases recorded in medical papers, "after a long illness A. died rather suddenly," or, "unexpectedly both to himself and to others." "Unexpectedly " to others, perhaps, who did not see, because they did not look; but by no means "unexpectedly to himself," as I feel entitled to believe, both from the internal evidence in such stories, and from watching similar cases: there was every reason to expect that A. would die, and he knew it; but he found it useless to insist upon his own knowledge to his friends.

In these remarks I am alluding neither to acute cases which terminate rapidly nor to "nervous" cases.

By the first much interest in their own danger is very rarely felt. In writings of fiction, whether novels or biographies, these death-beds are generally depicted as almost seraphic in lucidity of intelligence. Sadly large has been my experience in death-beds, and I can only say that I have seldom or never seen such. Indifference, excepting with regard to bodily suffering, or to some duty the dying man desires to perform, is the far more usual state.

The "nervous case," on the other hand, delights in f guring to himself and others a fictitious danger.

But the long chronic case, who knows too well himself, and who has been told by his physician that he will never enter active life again, who feels that every month he has to give up something he could do the month before—oh! spare such sufferers your chattering hopes. You do not know how you worry and weary them. Such real sufferers cannot bear to talk of themselves, still less to hope for what they cannot at all expect.

So also as to all the advice showered so profusely upon such sick, to leave off some occupation, to try some other doctor, some other house, climate, pill, powder, or specific; I say nothing of the inconsistency—for these advisers are sure to be the same persons who exhorted the sick man not to believe his own doctor's prognostics, because "doctors are always mistaken," but to believe some other doctor, because "this doctor is always right." Sure also are these advisers to be the persons to bring the sick man fresh occupation, while exhorting him to leave his own.

Wonderful is the face with which friends, lay and medical, will come in and worry the patient with recommendations to do something or other, having just as little knowledge as to its being feasible, or even safe for him, as if they were to recommend a man to take exercise, not knowing he had broken his leg. What would the friend say, if *he* were the medical attendant, and if the patient, because some *other* friend had come in, because somebody, anybody, nobody, had recommended something, anything, nothing, were to disregard *his* orders, and take that other body's recommendation? But people never think of this.

Wonderful presumption of the advisers of the sick.

A celebrated historical personage has related the common- Advisers the same now as two hundred years ago. places which, when on the eve of executing a remarkable reso- lution, were showered in nearly the same words by every one around successively for a period of six months. To these the personage states that it was found least trouble always to reply the same thing, viz., that it could not be supposed that such a resolution had been taken without sufficient previous consideration. To patients enduring every day for years from every friend or acquaintance, either by letter or *vivâ voce,* some torment of this kind, I would suggest the same answer. It would indeed be spared, if such friends and acquaintances would but consider for one moment, that it is probable the patient has heard such advice at least fifty times before, and that, had it been practicable, it would have been practised long ago. But of such consideration there appears to be no chance. Strange, though true, that people should be just the same in these things as they were a few hundred years ago!

To me these commonplaces, leaving their smear upon the cheerful, single-hearted, constant devotion to duty, which is so often seen in the decline of such sufferers, recall the slimy trail left by the snail on the sunny southern garden-wall loaded with fruit.

No mockery in the world is so hollow as the advice showered Mockery of the advice given to sick. upon the sick. It is of no use for the sick to say anything, for what the adviser wants is, *not* to know the truth about the state of the patient, but to turn whatever the sick may say to the support of his own argument, set forth, it must be repeated, without any inquiry whatever into the patient's real condition. "But it would be im- pertinent or indecent in me to make such an inquiry," says the adviser. True; and how much more impertinent is it to give your advice when you can know nothing about the truth, and admit you could not inquire into it.

To nurses I say—these are the visitors who do your patient harm. When you hear him told:—1. That he has nothing the matter with him, and that he wants cheering. 2. That he is com- mitting suicide, and that he wants preventing. 3. That he is the tool of somebody who makes use of him for a purpose. 4. That he will listen to nobody, but is obstinately bent upon his own way; and 5. That he ought to be called to the sense of duty, and is flying in the face of Providence;—then know that your patient is receiving all the injury that he can receive from a visitor.

How little the real sufferings of illness are known or understood. How little does any one in good health fancy him or even *her*self into the life of a sick person.

Do, you who are about the sick or who visit the sick, try and give Means of giving plea- sure to the sick. them pleasure, remember to tell them what will do so. How often in such visits the sick person has to do the whole conversation, exerting his own imagination and memory, while you would take the visitor, absorbed in his own anxieties, making no effort of memory or imagination, for the sick person. "Oh! my dear, I have so much to think of, I really quite forgot to tell him that; besides, I thought he would know it," says the visitor to another friend.. How could "he know it"? Depend upon it, the people who say this are really those who have little "to think of." There are many burthened with business who always manage to keep a pigeon-hole in their minds, full of things to tell the "invalid."

I do not say, don't tell him your anxieties—I believe it is good for him and good for you too; but if you tell him what is anxious, surely you can remember to tell him what is pleasant too.

A sick person does so enjoy hearing good news:—for instance, of a love and courtship, while in progress to a good ending. If you tell him only when the marriage takes place, he loses half the pleasure, which God knows he has little enough of; and ten to one but you have told him of some love-making with a bad ending.

A sick person also intensely enjoys hearing of any *material* good, any positive or practical success of the right. He has so much of books and fiction, of principles, and precepts, and theories; do, instead of advising him with advice he has heard at least fifty times before, tell him of one benevolent act which has really succeeded practically,—it is like a day's health to him.*

You have no idea what the craving of sick with undiminished power of thinking, but little power of doing, is to hear of good practical action, when they can no longer partake in it.

Do observe these things with the sick. Do remember how their life is to them disappointed and incomplete. You see them lying there with miserable disappointments, from which they can have no escape but death, and you can't remember to tell them of what would give them so much pleasure, or at least an hour's variety.

They don't want you to be lachrymose and whining with them, they like you to be fresh and active and interested, but they cannot bear absence of mind, and they are so tired of the advice and preaching they receive from every body, no matter whom it is, they see.

There is no better society than babies and sick people for one another. Of course you must manage this so that neither shall suffer from it, which is perfectly possible. If you think the "air of the sick room" bad for the baby, why it is bad for the invalid too, and, therefore, you will of course correct it for both. It freshens up a sick person's whole mental atmosphere to see "the baby." And a very young child, if unspoiled, will generally adapt itself wonderfully to the ways of a sick person, if the time they spend together is not too long.

If you knew how unreasonably sick people suffer from reasonable causes of distress, you would take more pains about all these things. An infant laid upon the sick bed will do the sick person, thus suffering, more good than all your logic. A piece of good news will do the same. Perhaps you are afraid of "disturbing" him. You say there is no comfort for his present cause of affliction. It is perfectly

* A small pet animal is often an excellent companion for the sick, for long chronic cases especially. A pet bird in a cage is sometimes the only pleasure of an invalid confined for years to the same room. If he can feed and clean the animal himself, he ought always to be encouraged to do so.

reasonable. The distinction is this, if he is obliged to act, do not "disturb" him with another subject of thought just yet; help him to do what he wants to do : but, if he *has* done this, or if nothing *can* be done, then "disturb" him by all means. You will relieve, more effectually, unreasonable suffering from reasonable causes by telling him "the news," showing him "the baby," or giving him something new to think of or to look at than by all the logic in the world.

It has been very justly said that the sick are like children in this, that there is no *proportion* in events to them. Now it is your business as their visitor to restore this right proportion for them—to shew them what the rest of the world is doing. How can they find it out otherwise ? You will find them far more open to conviction than children in this. And you will find that their unreasonable intensity of suffering from unkindness, from want of sympathy, &c., will disappear with their freshened interest in the big world's events. But then you must be able to give them real interests, not gossip.

NOTE.—There are two classes of patients which are unfortunately becoming more common every day, especially among women of the richer orders, to whom all these remarks are pre-eminently inapplicable. 1. Those who make health an excuse for doing nothing, and at the same time allege that the being able to do nothing is their only grief. 2. Those who have brought upon themselves ill-health by over pursuit of amusement, which they and their friends have most unhappily called intellectual activity. I scarcely know a greater injury that can be inflicted than the advice too often given to the first class "to vegetate"—or than the admiration too often bestowed on the latter class for "pluck." *Two new classes of patients peculiar to this generation.*

XIII. OBSERVATION OF THE SICK.

There is no more silly or universal question scarcely asked than this, "Is he better ?" Ask it of the medical attendant, if you please. But of whom else, if you wish for a real answer to your question, would you ask it? Certainly not of the casual visitor; certainly not of the nurse, while the nurse's observation is so little exercised as it is now. What you want are facts, not opinions—for who can have any opinion of any value as to whether the patient is better or worse, excepting the constant medical attendant, or the really observing nurse ? *What is the use of the question, Is he better ?*

The most important practical lesson that can be given to nurses is to teach them what to observe—how to observe—what symptoms indicate improvement—what the reverse—which are of importance—which are of none—which are the evidence of neglect—and of what kind of neglect.

All this is what ought to make part, and an essential part, of the training of every nurse. At present how few there are, either professional or unprofessional, who really know at all whether any sick person they may be with is better or worse.

The vagueness and looseness of the information one receives in answer to that much abused question, "Is he better ?" would be

[Original page no. 59]

ludicrous, if it were not painful. The only sensible answer (in the present state of knowledge about sickness) would be " How can I know ? I cannot tell how he was when I was not with him."

I can record but a very few specimens of the answers* which I have heard made by friends and nurses, and accepted by physicians and surgeons at the very bed-side of the patient, who could have contradicted every word, but did not—sometimes from amiability, often from shyness, oftenest from languor !

" How often have the bowels acted, nurse ? " " Once, sir." This generally means that the utensil has been emptied once, it having been used perhaps seven or eight times.

" Do you think the patient is much weaker than he was six weeks ago ? " " Oh no, sir; you know it is very long since he has been up and dressed, and he can get across the room now." This means that the nurse has not observed that whereas six weeks ago he sat up and occupied himself in bed, he now lies still doing nothing; that, although he can " get across the room," he cannot stand for five seconds.

Another patient who is eating well, recovering steadily, although slowly, from fever, but cannot walk or stand, is represented to the doctor as making no progress at all.

* It is a much more difficult thing to speak the truth than people commonly imagine. There is the want of observation *simple*, and the want of observation *compound*, compounded, that is, with the imaginative faculty. Both may equally intend to speak the truth. The information of the first is simply defective. That of the second is much more dangerous. The first gives, in answer to a question asked about a thing that has been before his eyes perhaps for years, information exceedingly imperfect, or says, he does not know. He has never observed. And people simply think him stupid.

The second has observed just as little, but imagination immediately steps in, and he describes the whole thing from imagination merely, being perfectly convinced all the while that he has seen or heard it; or he will repeat a whole conversation, as if it were information which had been addressed to him ; whereas it is merely what he has himself said to somebody else. This is the commonest of all. These people do not even observe that they have *not* observed nor remember that they have forgotten.

Courts of justice seem to think that any body can speak "the whole truth and nothing but the truth," if he does but intend it. It requires many faculties combined of observation and memory to speak " the whole truth " and to say " nothing but the truth."

" I knows I fibs dreadful : but believe me, Miss, I never finds out I have fibbed until they tells me so," was a remark actually made. It is also one of much more extended application than most people have the least idea of.

Concurrence of testimony, which is so often adduced as final proof, may prove nothing more, as is well known to those accustomed to deal with the unobservant imaginative, than that one person has told his story a great many times

I have heard thirteen persons "concur" in declaring that a fourteenth, who had never left his bed, went to a distant chapel every morning at seven o'clock.

I have heard persons in perfect good faith declare, that a man came to dine every day at the house where they lived, who had never dined there once ; that a person had never taken the sacrament, by whose side they had twice at least knelt at Communion ; that but one meal a day came out of a hospital kitchen, which for six weeks they had seen provide from three to five and six meals a day. Such instances might be multiplied *ad infinitum* if necessary.

Questions, too, as asked now (but too generally) of or about Leading ques-
patients, would obtain no information at all about them, even if the tions useless
person asked of had every information to give.. The question is or misleading.
generally a leading question; and it is singular that people never
think what must be the answer to this question before they ask
it: for instance, "Has he had a good night?" Now, one patient
will think he has a bad night if he has not slept ten hours without
waking. Another does not think he has a bad night if he has had
intervals of dosing occasionally. The same answer has actually been
given as regarded two patients—one who had been entirely sleepless
for five times twenty-four hours, and died of it, and another who had
not slept the sleep of a regular night, without waking. Why cannot
the question be asked, How many hours' sleep has —— had? and
at what hours of the night?* "I have never closed my eyes all
night," an answer as frequently made when the speaker has had
several hours' sleep as when he has had none, would then be less
often said. Lies, intentional and unintentional, are much seldomer
told in answer to precise than to leading questions. Another
frequent error is to inquire whether one cause remains, and not
whether the effect which may be produced by a great many different
causes, *not* inquired after, remains. As when it is asked, whether
there was noise in the street last night; and if there were not, the
patient is reported, without more ado, to have had a good night.
Patients are completely taken aback by these kinds of leading questions, and give only the exact amount of information asked for, even
when they know it to be completely misleading.. The shyness of
patients is seldom allowed for..

How few there are who, by five or six pointed questions, can
elicit the whole case and get accurately to know and to be able to
report *where* the patient is.

I knew a very clever physician, of large dispensary and hospital Means of
practice, who invariably began his examination of each patient with obtaining
"Put your finger where you be bad." That man would never waste inaccurate
his time with collecting inaccurate information from nurse or patient. information.
Leading questions always collect inaccurate information.

At a recent celebrated trial, the following leading question was
put successively to nine distinguished medical men. "Can you attribute these symptoms to anything else but poison?" And out of the
nine, eight answered "No!" without any qualification whatever. It
appeared, upon cross-examination :—1. That none of them had ever
seen a case of the kind of poisoning supposed. · 2. That none of them
had ever seen a case of the kind of disease to which the death, if not
to poison, was attributable.. 3. That none of them were even aware

---

* This is important, because on this depends what the remedy will be If a
patient sleeps two or three hours early in the night, and then does not sleep
again at all, ten to one it is not a narcotic he wants, but food or stimulus, or
perhaps only warmth. If on the other hand, he is restless and awake all night,
and is drowsy in the morning, he probably wants sedatives, either quiet, coolness,
or medicine, a lighter diet, or all four. Now the doctor should be told this, or
how can he judge what to give?

[Original page no. 61]

of the main fact of the disease and condition to which the death was attributable.

Surely nothing stronger can be adduced to prove what use leading questions are of, and what they lead to.

I had rather not say how many instances I have known, where, owing to this system of leading questions, the patient has died, and the attendants have been actually unaware of the principal feature of the case.

As to food patient takes or does not take.

It is useless to go through all the particulars; besides sleep, in which people have a peculiar talent for gleaning inaccurate information. As to food, for instance, I often think that most common question, How is your appetite? can only be put because the questioner believes the questioned has really nothing the matter with him, which is very often the case. But where there is, the remark holds good which has been made about sleep. The *same* answer will often be made as regards a patient who cannot take two ounces of solid food per diem, and a patient who does not enjoy five meals a day as much as usual.

Again, the question, How is your appetite? is often put when How is your digestion? is the question meant. No doubt the two things depend on one another. But they are quite different. Many a patient can eat, if you can only "tempt his appetite." The fault lies in your not having got him the thing that he fancies. But many another patient does not care between grapes and turnips,—everything is equally distasteful to him. He would try to eat anything which would do him good; but everything "makes him worse." The fault here generally lies in the cooking. It is not his "appetite" which requires "tempting," it is his digestion which requires sparing. And good sick cookery will save the digestion half its work.

There may be four different causes, any one of which will produce the same result, viz., the patient slowly starving to death from want of nutrition:

1. Defect in cooking;
2. Defect in choice of diet;
3. Defect in choice of hours for taking diet;
4. Defect of appetite in patient.

Yet all these are generally comprehended in the one sweeping assertion that the patient has "no appetite."

Surely many lives might be saved by drawing a closer distinction; for the remedies are as diverse as the causes. The remedy for the first is, to cook better; for the second, to choose other articles of diet; for the third, to watch for the hours when the patient is in want of food; for the fourth, to show him what he likes, and sometimes unexpectedly. But no one of these remedies will do for any other of the defects not corresponding with it.

I cannot too often repeat that patients are generally either too languid to observe these things, or too shy to speak about them; nor is it well that they should be made to observe them, it fixes their attention upon themselves.

[Original page no. 62]

Again, I say, what *is* the nurse or friend there for except to take note of these things, instead of the patient doing so ?*

Again, the question is sometimes put, Is there diarrhœa? And the answer will be the same, whether it is just merging into cholera, whether it is a trifling degree brought on by some trifling indiscretion, which will cease the moment the cause is removed, or whether there is no diarrhœa at all, but simply relaxed bowels. As to diarrhœa.

It is useless to multiply instances of this kind. As long as observation is so little cultivated as it is now, I do believe that it is better for the physician *not* to see the friends of the patient at all. They will oftener mislead him than not. And as often by making the patient out worse as better than he really is.

In the case of infants, *everything* must depend upon the accurate observation of the nurse or mother who has to report. And how seldom is this condition of accuracy fulfilled.

A celebrated man, though celebrated only for foolish things, has told us that one of his main objects in the education of his son, was to give him a ready habit of accurate observation, a certainty of perception, and that for this purpose one of his means was a month's course as follows:—he took the boy rapidly past a toy-shop; the father and son then described to each other as many of the objects as they could, which they had seen in passing the windows, noting them down with pencil and paper, and returning afterwards to verify their own accuracy. The boy always succeeded best, *e.g.*, if the father described 30 objects, the boy did 40, and scarcely ever made a mistake. Means of cultivating sound and ready observation.

I have often thought how wise a piece of education this would be for much higher objects; and in our calling of nurses the thing itself is essential. For it may safely be said, not that the habit of ready and correct observation will by itself make us useful nurses, but that without it we shall be useless with all our devotion.

I have known a nurse in charge of a set of wards who not only carried in her head all the little varieties in the diets which each patient was allowed to fix for himself, but also exactly what each patient had taken during each day. I have known another nurse in charge of one single patient, who took away his meals day after day all but untouched, and never knew it.

If you find it helps you to note down such things on a bit of paper, in pencil, by all means do so. I think it more often lames than strengthens the memory and observation. But if you cannot get the habit of observation one way or other, you had better give up the being a nurse, for it is not your calling, however kind and anxious you may be.

* It is commonly supposed that the nurse is there to spare the patient from making physical exertion for himself—I would rather say that she ought to be there to spare him from taking thought for himself. And I am quite sure, that if the patient were spared all thought for himself, and *not* spared all physical exertion, he would be infinitely the gainer. The reverse is generally the case in the private house. In the hospital it is the relief from all anxiety, afforded by the rules of a well-regulated institution, which has often such a beneficial effect upon the patient. More important to spare the patient thought than physical exertion.

Surely you can learn at least to judge with the eye how much an oz. of solid food is, how much an oz. of liquid. You will find this helps your observation and memory very much, you will then say to yourself "A. took about an oz. of his meat to day;" "B. took three times in 24 hours about ¼ pint of beef tea;" instead of saying "B. has taken nothing all day," or "I gave A. his dinner as usual."

Sound and ready observation essential in a nurse.

I have known several of our real old-fashioned hospital "sisters," who could, as accurately as a measuring glass, measure out all their patients' wine and medicine by the eye, and never be wrong. I do not recommend this, one must be very sure of one's self to do it. I only mention it, because if a nurse can by practice measure medicine by the eye, surely she is no nurse who cannot measure by the eye about how much food (in oz.) her patient has taken.* In hospitals those who cut up the diets give with quite sufficient accuracy, to each patient, his 12 oz. or his 6 oz. of meat without weighing. Yet a nurse will often have patients loathing all food and incapable of any will to get well, who just tumble over the contents of the plate or dip the spoon in the cup to deceive the nurse, and she will take it away without ever seeing that there is just the same quantity of food as when she brought it, and she will tell the doctor, too, that the patient

English women have great capacity of, but little practice in close observation.

* It may be too broad an assertion, and it certainly sounds like a paradox. But I think that in no country are women to be found so deficient in ready and sound observation as in England, while peculiarly capable of being trained to it. The French or Irish woman is too quick of perception to be so sound an observer— the Teuton is too slow to be so ready an observer as the English woman might be. Yet English women lay themselves open to the charge so often made against them by men, viz., that they are not to be trusted in handicrafts to which their strength is quite equal, for want of a practised and steady observation. In countries where women (with average intelligence certainly not superior to that of Englishwomen) are employed, e. g., in dispensing, men responsible for what these women do (not theorizing about man's and woman's "missions"), have stated that they preferred the service of women to that of men, as being more exact, more careful, and incurring fewer mistakes of inadvertence.

Now certainly Englishwomen are peculiarly capable of attaining to this.

I remember when a child, hearing the story of an accident, related by some one who sent two girls to fetch a "bottle of salvolatile from her room;" "Mary could not stir," she said, "Fanny ran and fetched a bottle that was not salvolatile, and that was not in my room."

Now this sort of thing pursues every one through life. A woman is asked to fetch a large new bound red book, lying on the table by the window, and she fetches five small old boarded brown books lying on the shelf by the fire. And this, though she has "put that room to rights" every day for a month perhaps, and must have observed the books every day, lying in the same places, for a month, if she had any observation.

Habitual observation is the more necessary, when any sudden call arises. If "Fanny" had observed "the bottle of salvolatile" in "the aunt's room," every day she was there, she would more probably have found it when it was suddenly wanted.

There are two causes for these mistakes of inadvertence. 1. A want of ready attention; only part of the request is heard at all. 2. A want of the habit of observation.

To a nurse I would add, take care that you always put the same things in the same places; you don't know how suddenly you may be called on some day to find something, and may not be able to remember in your haste where you yourself had put it, if your memory is not in the habit of seeing the thing there always.

has eaten all his diets as usual, when all she ought to have meant is that she has taken away his diets as usual.

Now what kind of a nurse is this?

I would call attention to something else, in which nurses frequently fail in observation. There is a well-marked distinction between the excitable and what I will call the *accumulative* temperament in patients. One will blaze up at once, under any shock or anxiety, and sleep very comfortably after it; another will seem quite calm and even torpid, under the same shock, and people say, "He hardly felt it at all," yet you will find him some time after slowly sinking. The same remark applies to the action of narcotics, of aperients, which, in the one, take effect directly, in the other not perhaps for twenty-four hours. A journey, a visit, an unwonted exertion, will affect the one immediately, but he recovers after it; the other bears it very well at the time, apparently, and dies or is prostrated for life by it. People often say how difficult the excitable temperament is to manage. I say how difficult is the *accumulative* temperament. With the first you have an out-break which you could anticipate, and it is all over. With the second you never know where you are—you never know when the consequences are over. And it requires your closest observation to know what *are* the consequences of what—for the consequent by no means follows immediately upon the antecedent—and coarse observation is utterly at fault.

Almost all superstitions are owing to bad observation, to the *post hoc, ergo propter hoc ;* and bad observers are almost all superstitious. Farmers used to attribute disease among cattle to witchcraft; weddings have been attributed to seeing one magpie, deaths to seeing three; and I have heard the most highly educated now-a-days draw consequences for the sick closely resembling these.

Another remark: although there is unquestionably a physiognomy of disease as well as of health; of all parts of the body, the face is perhaps the one which tells the least to the common observer or the casual visitor. Because, of all parts of the body, it is the one most exposed to other influences, besides health. And people never, or scarcely ever, observe enough to know how to distinguish between the effect of exposure, of robust health, of a tender skin, of a tendency to congestion, of suffusion, flushing, or many other things. Again, the face is often the last to shew emaciation. I should say that the hand was a much surer test than the face, both as to flesh, colour, circulation, &c., &c. It is true that there are *some* diseases which are only betrayed at all by something in the face, *e.g.*, the eye or the tongue, as great irritability of brain by the appearance of the pupil of the eye. But we are talking of casual, not minute, observation. And few minute observers will hesitate to say that far more untruth than truth is conveyed by the oft repeated words, He *looks* well, or ill, or better or worse.

Wonderful is the way in which people will go upon the slightest observation, or often upon no observation at all, or upon some *saw* which the world's experience, if it had any, would have pronounced utterly false long ago.

Difference of excitable and accumulative temperaments.

Superstition the fruit of bad observation.

Physionomy of disease little shewn by the face.

I have known patients dying of sheer pain, exhaustion, and want of sleep, from one of the most lingering and painful diseases known, preserve, till within a few days of death, not only the healthy colour of the cheek, but the mottled appearance of a robust child. And scores of times have I heard these unfortunate creatures assailed with, "I am glad to see you looking so well." "I see no reason why you should not live till ninety years of age." "Why don't you take a little more exercise and amusement?" with all the other commonplaces with which we are so familiar.

There is, unquestionably, a physiognomy of disease. Let the nurse learn it.

The experienced nurse can always tell that a person has taken a narcotic the night before by the patchiness of the colour about the face, when the re-action of depression has set in; that very colour which the inexperienced will point to as a proof of health.

There is, again, a faintness, which does not betray itself by the colour at all, or in which the patient becomes brown instead of white. There is a faintness of another kind which, it is true, can always be seen by the paleness.

But the nurse seldom distinguishes. She will talk to the patient who is too faint to move, without the least scruple, unless he is pale and unless, luckily for him, the muscles of the throat are affected and he loses his voice.

Yet these two faintnesses are perfectly distinguishable, by the mere countenance of the patient.

Peculiarities of patients.

Again, the nurse must distinguish between the idiosyncracies of patients. One likes to suffer out all his suffering alone, to be as little looked after as possible. Another likes to be perpetually made much of and pitied, and to have some one always by him. Both these peculiarities might be observed and indulged much more than they are. For quite as often does it happen that a busy attendance is forced upon the first patient, who wishes for nothing but to be "let alone," as that the second is left to think himself neglected.

Nurse must observe for herself increase of patient's weakness, patient will not tell her.

Again, I think that few things press so heavily on one suffering from long and incurable illness, as the necessity of recording in words from time to time, for the information of the nurse, who will not otherwise see, that he cannot do this or that, which he could do a month or a year ago. What is a nurse there for if she cannot observe these things for herself? Yet I have known—and known too among those—and *chiefly* among those—whom money and position put in possession of everything which money and position could give—I have known, I say, more accidents, (fatal, slowly or rapidly,) arising from this want of observation among nurses than from almost anything else. Because a patient could get out of a warm-bath alone a month ago—because a patient could walk as far as his bell a week ago, the nurse concludes that he can do so now. She has never observed the change; and the patient is lost from being left in a helpless state of exhaustion, till some one accidentally comes in. And this not from any unexpected apoplectic, paralytic, or fainting fit (though even these could be expected far more, at least, than they are now, if we did but *observe*). No, from the expected, or to be expected, inevitable, visible, calculable, uninterrupted increase of weakness, which none need fail to observe.

Again, a patient not usually confined to bed, is compelled by an attack of diarrhœa, vomiting, or other accident, to keep his bed for a few days; he gets up for the first time, and the nurse lets him go into another room, without coming in, a few minutes afterwards, to look after him. It never occurs to her that he is quite certain to be faint, or cold, or to want something. She says, as her excuse, Oh, he does not like to be fidgetted after. Yes, he said so some weeks ago; but he never said he did not like to be "fidgetted after," when he is in the state he is in now; and if he did, you ought to make some excuse to go in to him. More patients have been lost in this way than is at all generally known, viz., from relapses brought on by being left for an hour or two faint, or cold, or hungry, after getting up for the first time. *(margin: Accidents arising from the nurse's want of observation.)*

Yet it appears that scarcely any improvement in the faculty of observing is being made. Vast has been the increase of knowledge in pathology—that science which teaches us the final change produced by disease on the human frame—scarce any in the art of observing the signs of the change while in progress. Or, rather, is it not to be feared that observation, as an essential part of medicine, has been declining? *(margin: Is the faculty of observing on the decline.)*

Which of us has not heard fifty times, from one or another, a nurse, or a friend of the sick, aye, and a medical friend too, the following remark:—"So A is worse, or B is dead. I saw him the day before; I thought him so much better; there certainly was no appearance from which one could have expected so sudden (?) a change." I have never heard any one say, though one would think it the more natural thing, "There *must* have been *some* appearance, which I should have seen if I had but looked; let me try and remember what there was, that I may observe another time." No, this is not what people say. They boldly assert that there was nothing to observe, not that their observation was at fault.

Let people who have to observe sickness and death look back and try to register in their observation the appearances which have preceded relapse, attack, or death, and not assert that there were none, or that there were not the *right* ones.*

A want of the habit of observing conditions and an inveterate habit of taking averages are each of them often equally misleading. *(margin: Observation of general conditions.)*

* It falls to few ever to have had the opportunity of observing the different aspects which the human face puts on at the sudden approach of certain forms of death by violence; and as it is a knowledge of little use I only mention it here as being the most startling example of what I mean. In the nervous temperament the face becomes pale (this is the only *recognized* effect); in the sanguine temperament purple; in the bilious yellow, or every manner of colour in patches. Now, it is generally supposed that paleness is the one indication of almost any violent change in the human being, whether from terror, disease, or anything else. There can be no more false observation. Granted, it is the one recognized livery, as I have said—*de rigueur* in novels, but nowhere else. *(margin: Approach of death, paleness by no means an invariable effect, as we find in novels.)*

[Original page no. 67]

Men whose profession like that of medical men leads them to observe only, or chiefly, palpable and permanent organic changes are often just as wrong in their opinion of the result as those who do not observe at all. For instance, there is a broken leg; the surgeon has only to look at it once to know; it will not be different if he sees it in the morning to what it would have been had he seen it in the evening. And in whatever conditions the patient is, or is likely to be, there will still be the broken leg, until it is set. The same with many organic diseases. An experienced physician has but to feel the pulse once, and he knows that there is aneurism which will kill some time or other.

But with the great majority of cases, there is nothing of the kind; and the power of forming any correct opinion as to the result must entirely depend upon an enquiry into all the conditions in which the patient lives. In a complicated state of society in large towns, death, as every one of great experience knows, is far less often produced by any one organic disease than by some illness, after many other diseases, producing just the sum of exhaustion necessary for death. There is nothing so absurd, nothing so misleading as the verdict one so often hears: So-and-so has no organic disease,—there is no reason why he should not live to extreme old age; sometimes the clause is added, sometimes not: Provided he has quiet, good food, good air, &c., &c., &c.; the verdict is repeated by ignorant people *without* the latter clause; or there is no possibility of the conditions of the latter clause being obtained; and this, the *only* essential part of the whole, is made of no effect. I have heard a physician, deservedly eminent, assure the friends of a patient of his recovery. Why? Because he had now prescribed a course, every detail of which the patient had followed for years. And because he had forbidden a course which the patient could not by any possibility alter.*

* I have known two cases, the one of a man who intentionally and repeatedly displaced a dislocation, and was kept and petted by all the surgeons, the other of one who was pronounced to have nothing the matter with him, there being no organic change perceptible, but who died within the week. In both these cases, it was the nurse who, by accurately pointing out what she had accurately observed, to the doctors, saved the one case from persevering in a fraud, the other from being discharged when actually in a dying state.

I will even go further and say, that in diseases which have their origin in the feeble or irregular action of some function, and not in organic change, it is quite an accident if the doctor who sees the case only once a day, and generally at the same time, can form any but a negative idea of its real condition. In the middle of the day, when such a patient has been refreshed by light and air, by his tea, his beef tea, and his brandy, by hot bottles to his feet, by being washed and by clean linen, you can scarcely believe that he is the same person as lay with a rapid fluttering pulse, with puffed eye-lids, with short breath, cold limbs, and unsteady hands, this morning. Now what is a nurse to do in such a case? Not cry, " Lord bless you, sir, why you'd have thought he were a dying all night.". This may be true, but it is not the way to impress with the truth a doctor, more capable of forming a judgment from the facts, if he did but know them, than you are. What he wants is not your opinion, however respectfully given, but your facts. In all diseases it is important, but in diseases which do not run a distinct and fixed course, it is not only important, it is essential that the facts the nurse alone can observe, should be accurately observed, and accurately reported to the doctor.

Undoubtedly a person of no scientific knowledge whatever but of observation and experience in these kinds of conditions, will be able to arrive at a much truer guess as to the probable duration of life of members of a family or inmates of a house, than the most scientific physician to whom the same persons are brought to have their pulse felt; no enquiry being made into their conditions.

In Life Insurance and such like societies, were they instead of having the persons examined by a medical man, to have the houses, conditions, ways of life, of these persons examined, at how much truer results would they arrive! W. Smith appears a fine hale man, but it might be known that the next cholera epidemic he runs a bad chance. Mr. and Mrs. J. are a strong healthy couple, but it might be known that they live in such a house, in such a part of London, so near the river that they will kill four-fifths of their children; which of the children will be the ones to survive might also be known.

Averages again seduce us away from minute observation. "Average mortalities" merely tell that so many per cent. die in this town and so many in that, per annum. But whether A or B will be among these, the "average rate" of course does not tell. We know, say, that from 22 to 24 per 1,000 will die in London next year. But minute enquiries into conditions enable us to know that in such a district, nay, in such a street,—or even on one side of that street, in such a particular house, or even on one floor of that particular "Average rate of mortality" tells us only that so many per cent. will die. Observation must tell us *which* in the hundred they will be who will die.

I must direct the nurse's attention to the extreme variation there is not unfrequently in the pulse of such patients during the day. A very common case is this: Between 3 and 4 A.M. the pulse becomes quick, perhaps 130, and so thready it is not like a pulse at all, but like a string vibrating just underneath the skin. After this the patient gets no more sleep. About mid-day the pulse has come down to 80; and though feeble and compressible is a very respectable pulse. At night, if the patient has had a day of excitement, it is almost imperceptible. But, if the patient has had a good day, it is stronger and steadier and not quicker than at mid-day. This is a common history of a common pulse; and others, equally varying during the day, might be given. Now, in inflammation, which may almost always be detected by the pulse, in typhoid fever, which is accompanied by the low pulse that nothing will raise, there is no such great variation. And doctors and nurses become accustomed not to look for it. The doctor indeed cannot. But the variation is in itself an important feature.

Cases like the above often "go off rather suddenly," as it is called, from some trifling ailment of a few days, which just makes up the sum of exhaustion necessary to produce death. And everybody cries, who would have thought it? except the observing nurse, if there is one, who had always expected the exhaustion to come, from which there would be no rally, because she knew the patient had no capital in strength on which to draw, if he failed for a few days to make his barely daily income in sleep and nutrition.

I have often seen really good nurses distressed, because they could not impress the doctor with the real danger of their patient; and quite provoked because the patient "would look," either "so much better" or "so much worse" than he really is "when the doctor was there." The distress is very legitimate, but it generally arises from the nurse not having the power of laying clearly and shortly before the doctor the facts from which she derives her opinion, or from the doctor being hasty and inexperienced, and not capable of eliciting them. A man who really cares for his patients, will soon learn to ask for and appreciate the information of a nurse, who is at once a careful observer and a clear reporter.

house, will be the excess of mortality, that is, the person will die who ought not to have died before old age.

Now, would it not very materially alter the opinion of whoever were endeavouring to form one, if he knew that from that floor, of that house, of that street the man came.

Much more precise might be our observations even than this and much more correct our conclusions.

It is well known that the same names may be seen constantly recurring on workhouse books for generations. That is, the persons were born and brought up, and will be born and brought up, generation after generation, in the conditions which make paupers. Death and disease are like the workhouse, they take from the same family, the same house, or in other words the same conditions. Why will we not observe what they are?

The close observer may safely predict that such a family, whether its members marry or not, will become extinct; that such another will degenerate morally and physically. But who learns the lesson? On the contrary, it may be well known that the children die in such a house at the rate of 8 out of 10; one would think that nothing more need be said; for how could Providence speak more distinctly? yet nobody listens, the family goes on living there till it dies out, and then some other family takes it. Neither would they listen "if one rose from the dead."

What observation is for. In dwelling upon the vital importance of *sound* observation, it must never be lost sight of what observation is for. It is not for the sake of piling up miscellaneous information or curious facts, but for the sake of saving life and increasing health and comfort. The caution may seem useless, but it is quite surprising how many men (some women do it too), practically behave as if the scientific end were the only one in view, or as if the sick body were but a reservoir for stowing medicines into, and the surgical disease only a curious case the sufferer has made for the attendant's special information. This is really no exaggeration. You think, if you suspected your patient was being poisoned, say, by a copper, kettle, you would instantly, as you ought, cut off all possible connection between him and the suspected source of injury, without regard to the fact that a curious mine of observation is thereby lost. But it is not everybody who does so, and it has actually been made a question of medical ethics, what should the medical man do if he suspected poisoning? The answer seems a very simple one,—insist on a confidential nurse being placed with the patient, or give up the case.

What a confidential nurse should be. And remember every nurse should be one who is to be depended upon, in other words, capable of being a "confidential" nurse. She does not know how soon she may find herself placed in such a situation; she must be no gossip, no vain talker; she should never answer questions about her sick except to those who have a right to ask them; she must, I need not say, be strictly sober and honest; but more than this, she must be a religious and devoted woman; she must have a respect for her own calling;

because God's precious gift of life is often literally placed in her hands; she must be a sound, and close, and quick observer; and she must be a woman of delicate and decent feeling.

To return to the question of what observation is for:—It would really seem as if some had considered it as its own end, as if detection, not cure, was their business; nay more, in a recent celebrated trial, three medical men, according to their own account, suspected poison, prescribed for dysentery, and left the patient to the poisoner. This is an extreme case. But in a small way, the same manner of acting falls under the cognizance of us all. How often the attendants of a case have stated that they knew perfectly well that the patient could not get well in such an air, in such a room, or under such circumstances, yet have gone on dosing him with medicine, and making no effort to remove the poison from him, or him from the poison which they knew was killing him; nay, more, have sometimes not so much as mentioned their conviction in the right quarter —that is, to the only person who could act in the matter.

Observation is for practical purposes.

CONCLUSION.

The whole of the preceding remarks apply even more to children and to puerperal women than to patients in general. They also apply to the nursing of surgical, quite as much as to that of medical cases. Indeed, if it be possible, cases of external injury require such care even more than sick. In surgical wards, one duty of every nurse certainly is *prevention*. Fever, or hospital gangrene, or pyœmia, or purulent discharge of some kind may else supervene. Has she a case of compound fracture, of amputation, or of erysipelas, it may depend very much on how she looks upon the things enumerated in these notes, whether one or other of these hospital diseases attacks her patient or not. If she allows her ward to become filled with the peculiar close fœtid smell, so apt to be produced among surgical cases, especially where there is great suppuration and discharge, she may see a vigorous patient in the prime of life gradually sink and die where, according to all human probability, he ought to have recovered. The surgical nurse must be ever on the watch, ever on her guard, against want of cleanliness, foul air, want of light, and of warmth.

Sanitary nursing as essential in surgical as in medical cases, but not to supersede surgical nursing.

Nevertheless let no one think that because *sanitary* nursing is the subject of these notes, therefore, what may be called the handicraft of nursing is to be undervalued. A patient may be left to bleed to death in a sanitary palace. Another who cannot move himself may die of bed-sores, because the nurse does not know how to change and clean him, while he has every requisite of air, light, and quiet. But nursing, as a handicraft, has not been treated of here for three reasons: 1. that these notes do not pretend to be a manual for nursing, any more than for cooking for the sick; 2. that the writer, who has herself seen more of what may be called surgical nursing, *i. .e.* practical manual nursing, than, perhaps, any one in Europe,

[Original page no. 71]

honestly believes that it is impossible to learn it from any book, and that it can only be thoroughly learnt in the wards of a hospital; and she also honestly believes that the perfection of surgical nursing may be seen practised by the old-fashioned "Sister" of a London hospital, as it can be seen nowhere else in Europe. 3. While thousands die of foul air, &c., who have this surgical nursing to perfection, the converse is comparatively rare.

Children : their greater susceptibility to the same things.

To revert to children. They are much more susceptible than grown people to all noxious influences. They are affected by the same things, but much more quickly and seriously, viz., by want of fresh air, of proper warmth, want of cleanliness in house, clothes, bedding, or body, by startling noises, improper food, or want of punctuality, by dulness and by want of light, by too much or too little covering in bed, or when up, by want of the spirit of management generally in those in charge of them.   One can, therefore, only press the importance, as being yet greater in the case of children, greatest in the case of sick children, of attending to these things.

That which, however, above all, is known to injure children seriously is foul air, and most seriously at night. Keeping the rooms where they sleep tight shut up, is destruction to them.   And, if the child's breathing be disordered by disease, a few hours only of such foul air may endanger its life, even where no inconvenience is felt by grown-up persons in the same room.

The following passages, taken out of an excellent "Lecture on Sudden Death in Infancy and Childhood," just published, show the vital importance of careful nursing of children.   "In the great majority of instances, when death suddenly befalls the infant or young child, it is an *accident;* it is not a necessary, inevitable result of any disease from which it is suffering."

It may be here added, that it would be very desirable to know how often death is, with adults, "not a necessary, inevitable result of any disease."   Omit the word "sudden;" (for *sudden* death is comparatively rare in middle age ;) and the sentence is almost equally true for all ages.

The following causes of "accidental" death in sick children are enumerated :—"Sudden noises, which startle—a rapid change of temperature, which chills the surface, though only for a moment —a rude awakening from sleep—or even an over-hasty, or an over-full meal"—" any sudden impression on the nervous system—any hasty alteration of posture—in short, any cause whatever by which the respiratory process may be disturbed."

It may again be added, that, with very weak adult patients, these causes are also (not often "suddenly fatal," it is true, but) very much oftener than is at all generally known, irreparable in their consequences.

Both for children and for adults, both for sick and for well (although more certainly in the case of sick children than in any others), I would here again repeat, the most frequent and most fatal cause of all is sleeping, for even a few hours, much more for weeks and months, in foul air, a condition which, more than any other condition, disturbs the respiratory process, and tends to pro-duce "accidental" death in disease.

I need hardly here repeat the warning against any confusion of ideas between cold and fresh air. You may chill a patient fatally without giving him fresh air at all. And you can quite well, nay, much better, give him fresh air without chilling him. This is the test of a good nurse.

In cases of long recurring faintnesses from disease, for instance, especially disease which affects the organs of breathing, fresh air to the lungs, warmth to the surface, and often (as soon as the patient can swallow) hot drink, these are the right remedies and the only ones. Yet, oftener than not, you see the nurse or mother just reversing this; shutting up every cranny through which fresh air can enter, and leaving the body cold, or perhaps throwing a greater weight of clothes upon it, when already it is generating too little heat.

"Breathing carefully, anxiously, as though respiration were a function which required all the attention for its performance," is cited as a not unusual state in children, and as one calling for care in all the things enumerated above. That breathing becomes an almost voluntary act, even in grown up patients who are very weak, must often have been remarked.

"Disease having interfered with the perfect accomplishment of the respiratory function, some sudden demand for its complete exer-cise, issues in the sudden stand still of the whole machinery," is given as one process :—" life goes out for want of nervous power to keep the vital functions in activity," is given as another, by which " acci-dental" death is most often brought to pass in infancy.

Also in middle age, both these processes may be seen ending in death, although generally not suddenly. And I have seen, even in middle age, the " *sudden* stand-still" here mentioned, and from the same causes.

To sum up :—the answer to two of the commonest objections Summary. urged, one by women themselves, the other by men, against the desirableness of sanitary knowledge for women, *plus* a caution, comprises the whole argument for the art of nursing.

(1.) It is often said by men, that it is unwise to teach women Reckless ama-anything about these laws of health, because they will take to teur physick-physicking,—that there is a great deal too much of amateur physick- ing by women. ing as it is, which is indeed true. One eminent physician told me ledge of the that he had known more calomel given, both at a pinch and for a laws of health continuance, by mothers, governesses, and nurses, to children than alone can he had ever heard of a physician prescribing in all his experience. check this. Another says, that women's only idea in medicine is calomel and aperients. This is undeniably too often the case. There is nothing ever seen in any professional practice like the reckless physicking by amateur females.* But this is just what the really experienced and

* I have known many ladies who, having once obtained a " blue pill" prescrip- Danger of phy-tion from a physician, gave and took it as a common aperient two or three times sicking by a week—with what effect may be supposed. In one case I happened to be the amateur person to inform the physician of it, who substituted for the prescription a com- females.

[Original page no. 73]

observing nurse does *not* do; she neither physics herself nor others. And to cultivate in things pertaining to health observation and experience in women who are mothers, governesses or nurses, is just the way to do away with amateur physicking, and if the doctors did but know it, to make the nurses obedient to them,—helps to them instead of hindrances. Such education in women would indeed diminish the doctor's work—but no one really believes that doctors wish that there should be more illness, in order to have more work.

What pathology teaches. What observation alone teaches. What medicine does. What nature alone does.

(2.) It is often said by women, that they cannot know anything of the laws of health, or what to do to preserve their children's health, because they can know nothing of "Pathology," or cannot "dissect," —a confusion of ideas which it is hard to attempt to disentangle. Pathology teaches the harm that disease has done. But it teaches nothing more. We know nothing of the principle of health, the positive of which pathology is the negative, except from observation and experience. And nothing but observation and experience will teach us the ways to maintain or to bring back the state of health. It is often thought that medicine is the curative process. It is no such thing; medicine is the surgery of functions, as surgery proper is that of limbs and organs. Neither can do anything but remove obstructions; neither can cure; nature alone cures. Surgery removes the

paratively harmless aperient pill. The lady came to me and complained that it "did not suit her half so well."

If women will take or give physic, by far the safest plan is to send for "the doctor" every time—for I have known ladies who both gave and took physic, who would not take the pains to learn the names of the commonest medicines, and confounded, *e. g.*, colocynth with colchicum. This is playing with sharp edged tools "with a vengeance."

There are excellent women who will write to London to their physician that there is much sickness in their neighbourhood in the country, and ask for some prescription from him, which they used to like themselves, and then give it to all their friends and to all their poorer neighbours who will take it. Now, instead of giving medicine, of which you cannot possibly know the exact and proper application, nor all its consequences, would it not be better if you were to persuade and help your poorer neighbours to remove the dung-hill from before the door, to put in a window which opens, or an Arnott's ventilator, or to cleanse and lime-wash the cottages? Of these things the benefits are sure. The benefits of the inexperienced administration of medicines are by no means so sure.

Homœopathy has introduced one essential amelioration in the practice of physic by amateur females; for its rules are excellent, its physicking comparatively harmless—the "globule" is the one grain of folly which appears to be necessary to make any good thing acceptable. Let then women, if they will give medicine, give homœopathic medicine. It won't do any harm.

An almost universal error among women is the supposition that everybody *must* have the bowels opened once in every twenty-four hours or must fly immediately to aperients. The reverse is the conclusion of experience.

This is a doctor's subject, and I will not enter more into it; but will simply repeat, do not go on taking or giving to your children your abominable "courses of aperients," without calling in the doctor.

It is very seldom indeed, that by choosing your diet, you cannot regulate your own bowels; and every woman may watch herself to know what kind diet will do this; I have known deficiency of meat produce constipation, quite as often as deficiency of vegetables; baker's bread much oftener than either. Home made brown bread will oftener cure it than anything else.

bullet out of the limb, which is an obstruction to cure, but nature heals the wound. So it is with medicine; the function of an organ becomes obstructed ; medicine, so far as we know, assists nature to remove the obstruction, but does nothing more. And what nursing has to do in either case, is to put the patient in the best condition for nature to act upon him. Generally, just the contrary is done. You think fresh air, and quiet and cleanliness extravagant, perhaps dangerous, luxuries, which should be given to the patient only when quite convenient, and medicine the *sine quâ non*, the panacea. If I have succeeded in any measure in dispelling this illusion, and in showing what true nursing is, and what it is not, my object will have been answered.

Now for the caution :—

(3.) It seems a commonly received idea among men and even among women themselves that it requires nothing but a disappointment in love, the want of an object, a general disgust, or incapacity for other things, to turn a woman into a good nurse.

This reminds one of the parish where a stupid old man was set to be schoolmaster because he was " past keeping the pigs."

Apply the above receipt for making a good nurse to making a good servant. And the receipt will be found to fail.

Yet popular novelists of recent days have invented ladies disappointed in love or fresh out of the drawing-room turning into the war-hospitals to find their wounded lovers, and when found, forthwith abandoning their sick-ward for their lover, as might be expected. Yet in the estimation of the authors, these ladies were none the worse for that, but on the contrary were heroines of nursing.

What cruel mistakes are sometimes made by benevolent men and women in matters of business about which they can know nothing and think they know a great deal.

The everyday management of a large ward, let alone of a hospital —the knowing what are the laws of life and death for men, and what the laws of health for wards—(and wards are healthy or unhealthy, mainly according to the knowledge or ignorance of the nurse)—are not these matters of sufficient importance and difficulty to require learning by experience and careful inquiry, just as much as any other art? They do not come by inspiration to the lady disappointed in love, nor to the poor workhouse drudge hard up for a livelihood.

And terrible is the injury which has followed to the sick from such wild notions!

In this respect (and why is it so ?), in Roman Catholic countries, both writers and workers are, in theory at least, far before ours. They would never think of such a beginning for a good working Superior or Sister of Charity. And many a Superior has refused to admit a *Postulant* who appeared to have no better " vocation " or reasons for offering herself than these.

It is true *we* make " no vows." But is a " vow " necessary to convince us that the true spirit for learning any art, most especially an art of charity, aright, is not a disgust to everything or something else? Do we really place the love of our kind (and of nursing, as one branch of it,) so low as this? What would the Mère Angélique of Port Royal, what would our own Mrs. Fry have said to this?

NOTE.—I would earnestly ask my sisters to keep clear of both the jargons now current everywhere (for they *are* equally jargons); of the jargon, namely, about the "rights" of women, which urges women to do all that men do, including the medical and other professions, merely because men do it, and without regard to whether this *is* the best that women can do; and of the jargon which urges women to do nothing that men do, merely because they are women, and should be "recalled to a sense of their duty as women," and because "this is women's work," and "that is men's," and "these are things which women should not do," which is all assertion and nothing more. Surely woman should bring the best she has, *whatever* that is, to the work of God's world, without attending to either of these cries. For what are they, both of them, the one *just* as much as the other, but listening to the "what people will say," to opinion, to the "voices from without?" And as a wise man has said, no one has ever done anything great or useful by listening to the voices from without.

You do not want the effect of your good things to be, "How wonderful for a *woman!*" nor would you be deterred from good things, by hearing it said, "Yes, but she ought not to have done this, because it is not suitable for a woman." But you want to do the thing that is good, whether it is "suitable for a woman" or not.

It does not make a thing good, that it is remarkable that a woman should have been able to do it. Neither does it make a thing bad, which would have been good had a man done it, that it has been done by a woman.

Oh, leave these jargons, and go your way straight to God's work, in simplicity and singleness of heart.